UNDERSTANDING KETAMINE

SCIENCE, HISTORY, & A PATIENT'S JOURNEY TO
THE BOUNDARIES OF PSYCHEDELICS

The first educational memoir by

D. LAMAR

1

This book is dedicated to my Uncle Roger. Thank you for sticking by me through the darkest days, and encouraging me to write.

And to my mother, I love you.

Thank you to everyone who doubted me, for providing the limitless fuel required to write these words.

Copyright © 2022 Rain Media

All rights reserved. No part of this book may be reproduced, stored, or transmitted by any means. Neither auditory, graphic, mechanical, or electronic is permitted without written permission of the author, except in the case of brief excerpts used in critical articles and reviews. Unauthorized reproduction of any part of this book is illegal and is punishable by law. Cover design by ebooklaunch.com.

None of the contents of this book or related materials are to be taken as medical advice. This text and related materials DO NOT condone illegal activity, neither state nor federal. Consult a licensed medical provider for help.

ISBN: 979-8-9868193-0-3 (paperback)

ISBN: 979-8-9868193-1-0 (digital)

TABLE OF CONTENTS

FOREWORD 7

START HERE 10

1 HOW TO WIN 14

2 ALL YOUR PAIN IS FOR A PURPOSE 23

3 THE SETUP 36

4 WHAT IS KETAMINE AND WHAT ARE THE SIDE EFFECTS 56

5 A DRAMATIC HISTORY 64

6 HOW DOES IT WORK 68

7 WHAT ABOUT IT WORK 74

8 WHAT ABOUT THE OTHERS 81

9 LIFT OFF 89

10 WHAT DOES A KETAMINE INFUSION FEEL LIKE ... 96

11 THE RESULT 110

12 INTEGRATION	119
13 THINGS TO CONSIDER BEFORE GETTING A KETAMINE INFUSION	134
REFERENCES	147
AUTHOR'S NOTE	149
RESOURCES	151

FOREWORD

When I started working in the field of psychedelic science, most people would only know Ketamine to be a horse tranquilizer. Today, we know that Ketamine is not only a strong and safe anesthetic for humans, but in sub-anesthetic doses under a suitable set and setting, it can induce psychedelic experiences.

But what exactly are psychedelic experiences? The word derives from the Greek words psyche "mind" and delos "to manifest." These can be beautiful experiences of unity and love, but they can also be very challenging and difficult to integrate. In any case, psychedelic experiences can change the perspective on your environment, emotions, and belief system, even long after the pharmacological effects have passed.

There is a growing body of evidence on the safety and efficacy of psychedelics, and their therapeutic potential. It is important to remember; these substances were once discovered and implemented in psychiatry before they became illegal and stigmatized for political gain.

Daniel Lamar's Book Understanding Ketamine goes beyond understanding the pharmacological properties of the substance. He shares his journey from being diagnosed with several psychiatric disorders to a state of well-being. Through his book, you will understand how crucial therapeutic guidance and integration are when challenges arise, and how psychedelic substances like psilocybin, LSD, Ketamine, and MDMA do more than change your neurobiology; they are catalysts for transformation. It is not the substance that will do the changing ... it is you.

Currently, most of these substances are illegal and unavailable in medical care. Ketamine, on the other hand, is legal and well-studied to have positive effects. It is, however, only human to forget the tools we have available right now and trick ourselves into thinking, "if only we had psychedelic mushrooms available, then we'd be able to end the mental health crisis," instead of taking action and further developing the tools already at our disposition to generate more significant effects.

As one of the founders and medical director of the first psychedelic clinic in Germany, I've seen how the field has developed through the years. I still remember how we decided to open the first clinic. After working for several years as MIND Academy director at the MIND Foundation, we thought the time was right to not only build research and educational programs for professionals and the general public, but also to put theory into practice and create forms of therapy for those that need solutions now. Using Ketamine and other non-pharmacological methods, we induce psychedelic experiences, which can lead to long-lasting effects beyond mere pharmacology when integrated with a psychotherapeutic context.

Mr. Lamar's book is being published with very appropriate timing. It provides people interested in this field with a balanced and informed patient perspective on what we can expect from this innovation in the future, and what is already available for those without the luxury of being able to wait.

Sergio Pérez Rosal, MD.
CEO and Medical Director of OVID Clinics | Board MBR of the MIND Foundation, Europe

START HERE

I'm always puzzled when society assumes understanding, especially with topics as complex as this. Sometimes this can be chalked up to intellectual laziness, and other times the opposite. Let's take a look at the word "fear" as an example of a malleable definition.

Fear can show up alongside many emotions and circumstances. Some people use it as a shield to repel risk. For example, someone may say, "I'm afraid to start a business because I might go broke." Sometimes people use fear as an excuse to quit — it's such a reliable escape valve for quitters. You don't need to be afraid of a clown in a sewer to be strangled by fear. Time, as my teacher, showed me how to look at fear differently.

Fear is always present in us. It's essential to the human condition. Without fear, there is no bravery. Without bravery, there are no hunters. Without hunters, there is no food. The world relies on fear to function. Those who can harness it, who can tame it, are essential to our survival as a species, and for future development. You get to decide which one you'll be: a lion tamer, or prey. You don't have to worry about deciding now, because this evolutionary puzzle piece is always hovering above us, forever malleable and just waiting to be placed and secured in time. Fear tumbles effortlessly alongside human development, creating the outputs of our evolution by naturally selecting the winners and the losers.

I'm afraid of belly-flopping on a fifty-foot cliff dive, but I'll never avoid the jump. I'm afraid of getting my nose broken, but I always stand up for myself; if I punch first, then I punch twice. I'm afraid of getting stabbed, but if you were my girlfriend, I'd embrace a blade to keep a scratch from touching your skin. I'd rather get shot, though (just an FYI).

What are you more afraid of — the fear itself, or the actions required to overcome it?

I fear failing at writing this book, but I'm willing to walk through the consequences of spending money and time to make it come alive. I know I will miss 100 percent of the swings I don't take. This is the difference between fear and being afraid. Being afraid is being stuck and not moving. Being in fear is the signal of power to come; the signal for action.

I am only enthusiastic to conquer fears I consider "worth it." It's good that I'm not the one who decides. I'm not the one controlling the signals. Whoever does places a lot of hard things in my path. I fall down and get banged up a few times, and then I get back up and tackle whatever is in my way. That's what we do, me and this invisible force. Some call it God, or the universe. I call it a partnership — though I don't get to make the big decisions, and I'm never the teacher.

The marriage of fear, action, and God fuels many of the best minds in the world. What is the difference between them and everyone else? Successful people choose to walk through the fear while others stay scared. If you stay scared, you stay low value. But if you are willing to walk through fear, then you will watch fire forge your mind's iron and suck out impurities in real time. Everyone is afraid, but not everyone is willing. What is truly terrifying, is the absence of action.

Whenever I go through something difficult or want to create something challenging, I lean on this side of myself. And I suggest you do, too. It is likely stronger than you think. When I'm comfortable, I'm lazy, forgetting fear can be morphed into fuel for maneuvering the jagged corners of life.

Fear is the signal for growth and green lights. What follows is likely to define us. If you quit, it can also be life-defining in another way.

> *"Extinguish the spark of fear with the fire of courage."*
>
> *— ANONYMOUS*

Everything you know about fear is fake. And, everything I knew about psychedelics was wrong. This is Understanding Ketamine.

1

HOW TO WIN

Some names, locations, and details have been changed in this book to protect the identity of others. Is that a shitty first sentence? Now I've asked a question, cursed, and led with meaningless garbage — all three big writing "no-no's" broken in the first paragraph. Excellent, Daniel, excellent. My writing mentor would say cursing in a book is oftentimes a sign of intellectual negligence, veiled in authenticity. "Swearing is an easy cop-out to using a more descriptive word or phrase," he'd say. I've been breaking the rules since I could read. Perhaps that's why I decided to become an author.

This memoir/educational hybrid is intended to educate on new psychedelic approaches to hard-to-treat mental health conditions otherwise failed by traditional medicine. A memoir is what people in writing circles call a story about an author's life. I start with broad information and history on psychedelics, then narrow it down into my experience using ketamine under a provider's care to treat depression and anxiety. In order for me to educate you, you will need to trust me. This is where it gets tricky. I am not a PhD, nor am I a perfect human. But because I have trudged through more horrific events in life to count, and subsequently studied mental health and psychedelics for the better part of a decade, the consecutive learnings have left a permanent tattoo on my to-do list: it's time to pass on the education to you.

I am not trying to sell you. This is either a win-win or lose-lose situation. We both win if you learn, and lose if you don't. In order to win, you will need to be an ideal student, sucking all the sweet psychoactive nectar from these pages. In order to be an ideal student, you'll need some degree of trust in me. Imagine hiring a basketball coach who always loses, or shoots granny style. No thank you. You wouldn't trust him, and neither would I.

I read books to learn, and sometimes to be entertained. This book is intended to do both. Without a strong thought leader, execution, action, and focus are the mere afterthoughts of a failing formula of education. We will start small. I believe trust is earned and not given. In order to achieve this, I'm going to take risks of vulnerability, revealing truths on these pages no other soul has ever seen or heard. This is a risk for me. I'm qualified in this topic primarily because of my trauma. My upbringing was not easy. More on that later.

The greatest and most successful men always are forged into gold through fire, always through adversity. This is one of the greatest and most unmistakable forces of nature.

I've been carved into a savage through trauma, but I'm a successful professional, son, cousin, a business owner, scientific researcher, Bitcoin fanatic, and internet entrepreneur. My colleagues and my family will read these books. I have no idea how they are going to react to the level of vulnerability I'm willing to display. I show that vulnerability to not only earn your trust and educate you at an effortless pace, but so I can relate to you and you with me. The following pages will illuminate close-minded corners using a combination of research, data, and personal experience.

To be clear, let me break down the mission. If I can help 100 people with these intros into psychedelic medicine, I'll cut my heart out and slap it down right on the pages for everyone to see it. The goal is to help the reader, and I hope the words I choose are able to instill confidence in my desire to explore this life-changing topic with you in a way that's fruitful.

How you apply knowledge is called "integration." This is your job. Learn, integrate, repeat. And in exchange for my transparent bleedings on these pages, hopefully my colleagues and friends won't disown me. I've learned there is extreme power within those who are vulnerable and transparent. It is not a weakness. You know the saying: "Those who mind don't matter because those who matter don't mind."

Since making the decision to work for myself, I've been gifted the ability to travel. I've been all over the world, from Asia to South America. Outside of most countries in the Western world, I've observed a consistently strong reliance on psychoactive plants for mental and spiritual health. This pattern varies in substance, from ayahuasca in Peru, to mushrooms in Bali, to peyote in Mexico.

In virtually every region in South and Central America, Mexico, Africa and Southeast Asia, psychedelic plants are used for hard-to-treat mental health disorders like addiction and depression. Perhaps the most striking example is the use of ibogaine, a psychedelic African root bark. It is commonly used to treat severe opiate addiction, and it works incredibly well at interrupting opiate withdrawal. Ibogaine seems to potentially reset the brain, sending the user into a four-to-six-hour vision quest, helping them untangle problems which seemed impossible to unravel before.

The ibogaine user can walk into their experience fully addicted to heroin, and wake up six hours later without withdrawal symptoms. That should be impossible; at the very least, it's impossible to ignore. But somehow, we in the West historically do exactly that — we ignore it.

This is a 2 book series, starting with text primarily about ketamine. This is also a story about me. My personal experiences with psychedelics treating trauma of all kinds, help to demystify the scientific nature of the topic into something more digestible and easy to understand.

I already put in the work, so readers, relax. If you learn how these substances work, what they are, the pros and cons, and so on, then you will have an easier time deciding which options are available to explore in your personal search for solutions, even when those solutions are outside the sparse medical approaches we've historically settled for.

This new psychedelic wave is set to collide with hard-to-treat mental health problems using the force of God itself, and you deserve to be prepared. And if we do this together safely, and don't screw it up like the hippies of 1968, people's lives will be changed.

I've received almost all the diagnoses in-the-book: PTSD, generalized anxiety, substance use disorder, and the rapidly growing focus of ketamine, treatment-resistant depression (TRD). Treatment-resistant means, in simple terms, the group of people who've tried multiple depression medications and failed to get relief. These are my own experiences and not meant to be taken as medical advice. Don't break the law; keep your doctor looped in.

By the end of this book you'll know what ketamine is, how it's being used medically, and what it feels like to take it. The reason this book series starts with ketamine is because it's the only psychoactive chemical legally used today in the Western world for mental health. "Ketamine" is the most searched term on Google in the psychedelic genre, tripling in search volume over the last three years across every state in the country. Depending on the state, it's searched three to four times as often as the popular query "magic mushrooms." Psilocybin, the active psychedelic ingredient in mushrooms, will be medically legal in Oregon by January 2023. It will be used to remedy a host of conditions. This trend will likely flow similar to the marijuana legalization movement, starting with progressive states and creeping deeper into the conservative states until each one has tipped over, spilling into the largest attempted mental health 180 we may see in our lifetimes.

The psychoactive fungus is now close to legal status and the most popular in traditional media. I assume MDMA treatment for PTSD is to follow, but ketamine treatment for depression — with a doctor's supervision — is already here.

For 12 months straight, I underwent ketamine therapy with a provider to treat depression, attending 18 separate infusions. The word "infusion" means medicine administered via an IV. In ketamine's mental health approach, an infusion lasts around an hour. My doctor visits also birthed a year-long data set which reflects the treatment's results into easy-to-digest numbers. I decided to include my unscripted personal diary of my experiences inside the ketamine world. Wherever it is I was sent, it was a powerful place, where the limits of the mind are shattered into dust, never to solidify again. The diary entries used to recall the events are original, dated in italics, and placed throughout this book.

The currency I paid for the information in these pages was not monetary. I spent $9,000 on ketamine sessions,

$20,000 on ibogaine treatment in Mexico, and $2,000 on a trip to Peru's ayahuasca-infused jungles and back. But that is nothing. The excruciating, mind-numbing stress, substance dependence, PTSD, and depression was a mountain so high its crest sits among gods. I experienced such extreme isolation, loneliness in rooms full of people, and a pain so deep I can only pray I succeed in describing the soul-crushing prison of darkness I stumbled through to get here.

As you will see, I am not a perfect poster-child for psychedelic therapies. There are multiple reasons for this, some fault of my own and some not. I wrote the book anyway, knowing that if we waited for a perfect princess (who's also a writer) to conquer a lifetime of trauma with one approach, or one type of treatment, without mistakes or room for error, we could be waiting a lifetime. The impact of these treatments was incredibly powerful, but I am only a human; imperfect and full of mistakes. To expect these medicines to be a magic pill is very American. Even if they are revealed to be the best tools in the shed, they still require a holistic approach that was not available in any of the early stage treatments I received. If you are searching for perfection, or some sort of psychedelic savior, you can stop reading now. If you are like me, and appreciate a very real and honest approach, welcome home.

2

ALL YOUR PAIN IS FOR A PURPOSE

As I lay in the hospital with a brace around my neck, I looked down at my right arm. It was white, bloated, and hardly recognizable. Welcome to Christmas day. I slipped coming down the stairs in my house and cracked vertebrae in the thoracic section of my back. When I fell, I heard the pop. The internal sensation of cracking bones was in competition with the audible sound, and I couldn't tell which was louder ... the sound or the feeling of my back breaking. I instantly blacked out and couldn't move. I was still conscious, but I couldn't see. *I'm too young — an internet entrepreneur, a health freak ... I can't get hurt like this!* I thought.

About 90 seconds went by, and I was slowly able to move pieces of my body again. They came online one by one. First came my legs, and then my fingers and arms. My vision returned and I slowly rose to my feet. It was Christmas Eve, and I was heading to my mom's house to have dinner with the family and exchange gifts. I called her.

"Mom, I just fell and it didn't sound good. I blacked out for a while. I think I'm okay, but I just wanted to call someone and let them know. It didn't feel right."

"Did you relapse?" she said.

I started scanning my brain, searching for the appropriate answer to give. I wasn't "sober" like a twelve-step group would define it. I had been taking Valium and other anti-anxiety meds intermittently, sometimes prescribed and sometimes not, when I felt I needed it for anxiety flare-ups or sleep. At the same time, I was giving my best shot at recreational cocaine here and there. After all, I was spending a lot of time in Colombia back then.

"Yes, I did ...?" I said. I sat thinking to myself, *I just need to be honest with her. But she knows I'm not "sober," so why would she ask? I have lived the same way for over a decade, and although the previous weeks haven't been my best stretch, I was working through it as I'd learned to do.*

I don't think me not being straight-edge sober like when I was 24 years old had anything to do with my fall. I tried to piece it together. *It's 10 a.m. I'm not physically dependent or addicted to any substance, and I feel fine. I'm a little scared because that fall didn't feel right.*

When there is a history of substance dependency among relationships, it can create a PTSD-like recall scenario for the individuals involved. I had been walking in a shadow of regret for twelve years, while my mom just wanted it never to happen again.

She proceeded to go silent and then hung up the phone. *Why didn't she ask me any questions?* I thought. *She can't be mad at me for being honest with her about not being completely straight-edge sober — she already knew.*

I didn't get it. I hadn't been "sober" since my twenties, and it wasn't a secret, but rather a conscious choice. I didn't understand why she used the term "relapse." *I thought she knew.* I walked upstairs to continue getting ready, and boom — total and complete blackness.

I collapsed on my bedroom floor for approximately the next twenty hours with a concussion, an acute kidney injury, and a broken back. Folding over myself, I cut off the blood flow to my right arm almost completely. Everything I knew about myself, my work, my health, and my financial security abruptly dissolved in seconds.

When I woke up, I looked down at my arm and instantly knew something was wrong. The audible crack when falling was now the least of my concerns. I started driving myself to the hospital when I got a phone call from an anonymous good friend.

She's anonymous for the sake of preserving her personal reputation on these pages. I'll be broad. She was family.

"Where are you?" she said. "We've been trying to find you. I went to your house and knocked on the door but you didn't answer. I've been calling. What is going on?!" I told her my arm was hurt and I was on my way to the hospital. I was still woozy and confused about what was actually taking place.

"Do you know what day it is?" she said.

"Ummm, Christmas Eve?" I replied.

"No, dude, you are missing a day. It's Christmas!"

I went back to my house to meet and let her drive me to the hospital. It was a terrible idea for me to be driving a car. The pressure in my arm was building and it was starting to go numb. On top of the physical pain, my brain felt completely scrambled. It was a feeling I hadn't experienced before that day. When she arrived at my house, her face was made up of a combination of astonishment, fear, and relief. The emotions were all mixed together into one facial expression I decoded into the fact... she loved me.

For the first time I felt like I knew it, despite how hardened the outer shell she displayed. It's not like our relationship was bad. She was the type to not really talk about the hard stuff. And my life, up until this point, was made up of 90 percent hard stuff. It was impossible to ignore, but easy to sweep into the communicative denial pile in hopes of a normal, turbulence-free relationship.

I couldn't blame her. I'd lived through so much chaos in comparison it was uncomfortable for my family and some friends to talk to me, and for me to talk to them. My life was so far outside their personal boundaries and consequential view of normalcy. I was the person in the family with a drug-riddled father's side, and an often-incarcerated dad. I had past addiction problems myself, starting around age 18 to 24 when I became dependent on pills at the height of the OxyContin epidemic. I'd been to rehab in my twenties caused by an ongoing war with mental health obstacles.

I was the guy who'd had an anxiety attack and ended up in the hospital for three days after online regulators took my supplement business down. They said I was "trying to cure addiction" by selling a formula I'd developed for over two years. The formula included ingredients shown in studies to decrease cravings in those with an addicted past. What I thought was my life's purpose was taken in an instant. I was the guy with problems.

I was the person in the family who was raped in junior high by another guy who was much bigger than me; I never told another soul until the age of thirty. I was the guy who was constantly telling my family to buy Bitcoin at $6,000, and to turn off the news because it was only leveraging their fear in exchange for clicks and views. I was the guy who thought differently. I was the guy with problems.

My relationships were also shallow because I was afraid to be honest with my family. I was afraid that they would judge me for who I was. We didn't often talk about things that mattered, like love, compassion for others, acceptance, and spiritual growth. And considering I was the only person in my direct family who wasn't a Christian, that seemed ironic. Consequently, I was definitely qualified as a self-proclaimed outsider.

I hope I make my mom proud by writing this book, but I fear the vulnerability written in these pages. Being vulnerable to you, the reader, is easy — I don't know you. But bleeding on a page for all my loved ones to see, judge, or label is a risk that I'm willing to take if the contents in this book go on to crack otherwise sealed-shut minds, and highlight new options to minimize the suffering of others.

At the same time as having lots of trauma, however, I was the guy who built a booming online business. I was the first of my family to graduate from a university with a degree in anything. No one in my family had an education up until this point. I was proudly the benefactor of a full-ride scholarship from the best business school in the state after submitting two essays about my childhood experiences, mental-health hurdles, and hopes to achieve personal and professional success like my grandfather.

The university is highly competitive and does not give out full-ride scholarships to many people. By the end of my junior year, I'd earned two of them.

The fuel that drove me through college was derived from fear of being like my parents. I didn't want to go to prison like my dad. And although I admire and respect my mom's work ethic, I didn't want to work 24/7 in a cubicle like her.

I'm leaving a lot of details about my father out of this book. When one has suffered the pain at a level so high most others in the population can't compute it, there are things worth keeping buried to just rest. The bottom line is this: I certainly did have "problems," but in my heart I knew that I had a powerful drive to do something important. I wasn't like everyone else, but I never wanted to be like them anyway.

When my friend and I arrived at the hospital, the doctors took one look at my arm and told me that I'd need surgery right away or I'd lose it. They also said my kidneys were failing because the muscle cells in my arm were dying, sending signals to the kidneys to turn off. As I looked at my bloated arm that day, the surgeon came in and explained I had compartment syndrome, and that the surgery I was about to undergo was the most painful surgery there was. It was literally number one on the charts.

I didn't have a choice. "Okay," I said.

"When you fell, were you under the influence?" he asked.

"I don't think so," I said. "I remember it very clearly and I hadn't taken anything yesterday when I slipped. But I'd taken some Valium the day before and was dabbling in some pretty strong Colombian cocaine this month. I suppose some of the after-effects may have affected my balance coming down the stairs." I continued, "I've had a problem with opiates in the past. My pain tolerance is very low, but I don't want to leave here dependent physically on opiates again. Consider the options when prescribing meds to me."

Even though I hadn't been using opiates leading up to the accident, the previous use had affected my pain tolerance. The doctor acknowledged my concern, but in my heart I knew I was screwed. *There's no way I'm getting out of this hospital without a good old-fashioned drug dependence problem,* I thought. The fear creeping in of the unavoidable withdrawals haunted my mind. And for the first time since I fell, I was afraid.

Ten days, three surgeries, and seven incisions later, my arm got infected in the hospital. Another surgery was ordered to fix it. My arm and hand were so swollen from compartment syndrome that they couldn't sew them shut. Three of the seven incisions would heal open without stitches or staples. The reason for the infection was simple. My forearm was split wide open, about 6 inches long and 2 inches wide, like a wedged chunk chopped out the side of a watermelon.

My hand had two open wounds. On the karate chop side of my hand, under my pinky, was a 1.5-inch-long and half-inch-wide open incision. On the other end of the same hand below my thumb was a 2x2-inch gaping hole that burned as if a hot blade was resting on my muscle tissue. It was graphic, and to this day the photos are hard for me to look at. As I constantly bled through the bandages, the staff cleaned and rewrapped them daily. Rubber bands were used in place of staples or stitches to hold the skin from stretching any further apart than it already was. Because of the uncontrolled inflammation of muscle tissue minimizing stitching ability, half the cuts would have to heal without stitches, open.

At this point, my back was the least of my worries. I was in a brace for a few days and it healed itself. My arm was the problem. I was in agonizing physical pain, and mentally I was having a hard time keeping it together. The Covid-19 virus was raging, so I could only choose one visitor. Since my anonymous friend brought me, she was the natural choice. She came to visit twice, but outside of that, I was alone. It was just me and my exposed muscle tissue … all day … all night.

Every day, the doctor would warn me that my kidneys were close to failing and I may need to go on dialysis. They forced me to eat certain foods and restricted my diet in hopes of bringing my kidneys back. It wasn't good. The anxiety was difficult to manage, and I had numerous bouts of breaking out into tears. I was alone. And as expected, the pain meds weren't working.

Throughout my two-week hospital stay, I graduated throughout the ranks of opiate medications, from morphine, to oxycodone, to Dilaudid, and then finally to intravenous fentanyl. Every 20 minutes, I would press a button and get a shot of the world's most deadly and rapidly addictive opiate flushed into my veins. Seven hundred mcgs every hour was the maximum dose prescribed. For those who don't know … that's a lot. It's approximately enough to kill five people without an opiate tolerance.

Three separate times, the hospital staff had to put a drug known as Narcan in my IV to counteract the fentanyl and keep my lungs working. I was on so much pain medicine they had to counteract it with another medication to increase the amount of breaths I was taking per minute. Otherwise, I may have died from lack of oxygen. When one is prescribed Narcan to go with their opiate prescription, you know you're playing a dangerous game — a balancing act only won if you don't die, and lost if you do.

Fentanyl has been widely blamed for reigniting the opioid epidemic and is responsible for more overdose deaths than heroin and meth combined. Its rapid onset and extreme affinity to the opioid receptors in the body make it one of the most effective painkillers on the planet, but also the most addictive and deadly.

Up until recently, if a heroin addict is put in jail, the medical staff will let him detox on a concrete slab with little to no medication. The withdrawal is extremely uncomfortable, but not deadly.

Opiates are notoriously agonizing to come off of, but it's very uncommon to die. Up until this point, the only drugs one commonly dies from in withdrawal are alcohol and Xanax (benzodiazepines). When fentanyl started showing up in heroin and fake blue oxycodone began flooding the streets, the state of the opiate epidemic came to a turning point. People started dropping like flies. Dying. Corpses lined the streets of my hometown city, slumped over with charred tinfoil in their hands. It looked like they were taking a nap after working the coal mines, only overdosed from smoking fentanyl-laced everything.

Fentanyl is so strong that heroin users even stopped using needles. They didn't have to anymore. Smoking fentanyl apparently is a better rush than shooting heroin. But there's a problem. For the first time in the drug war's history, people started dying from withdrawal of this newly popular synthetic opiate. Fentanyl was deadly enough in withdrawal to force even the jails to start updating their medical protocols.

In Washington and other states, they now treat addicts by weaning them off slowly instead of shaking it out on a bench with their black, charred fingers crossed. It's much more convenient for the jails this way: give the caged animals a few pills and the deputies don't have to scrape dead bodies off of their floors as often. After all, a dead inmate is not a profitable one.

Twenty-four-seven intravenous fentanyl every 20 minutes obviously worked for my pain. And the 4.5 mgs of Klonopin throughout the day took care of any anxiety I had over my exposed muscle tissues peeling from my arm like a fileted lobster tail. But my brain was like a mental torture chamber. Not only did I know that I wouldn't be able to work without typing, and I'd be at least temporarily disabled, but I was rapidly becoming dependent on the worst version of the drug I loved and hated the most, opiates.

The daily prescribed mix of Ativan, Klonopin, Xanax, and Valium would secure my dependence on benzodiazepines, the most deadly substance to come off of next to alcohol because of the seizure risk. When people stop taking benzos, they have seizures and die. When some people stop taking fentanyl, they also die. I sat in the hospital on those last days, now physically addicted to two substances that had potentially deadly consequences upon cessation. It took a moment to register the pain that was undoubtedly to come whenever I'd be required to come off of these medications. And during those last days, I remembered something I was "told" a year before, during an infusion of the powerful and prescribed psychedelic, ketamine.

"Son. All your pain, all of it, is for a purpose."

3

THE SETUP

Before you read any further, I need to preface a critically important point. If you don't understand all of what I'm about to say in these few sentences, stick with me. I will cover it all in the upcoming pages. You need to know, this is not a story of a mistake-free victory conquering mental health. Yes, you read the last chapter right. Regrettably, I did use illicit drugs a few times, even after my treatments. Despite the gravity of ketamine therapy, which I can't tell you about quite yet without ruining the story, life still happens. After surviving the nightmare I touched on in the last chapter, I made the decision to live sober from any narcotics with addiction potential...although I am not from the camp who believes all drugs are inherently negative. They are tools, which can be used for good and bad - consider OxyContin - it's a great pain killer, but it causes a lot of destruction when abused. In my case, because of my difficult history with substances as a younger man, using any drugs at all was a bad call. It would've been nice to undergo treatment and be perfect from that point on. But that wasn't my reality.

Many people will say, "If ketamine worked so well then why did you still play around with drugs afterward?" My response to that is simple but critically important — come to think of it, this alone may be THE MOST IMPORTANT POINT OF THIS BOOK. Ketamine and psychedelics are not a cure-all, nor do they treat every single type of mental health diagnosis equally. People will seek help with psychedelics like ketamine to treat depression, but many of them will have other chronic issues to tackle. Imagine treating a headache with aspirin and expecting it to also address your sinus infection ... doesn't make a lot of sense. Ketamine is being studied to minimize substance use disorder and PTSD symptoms, but overall the jury is still out. Both of which I have been diagnosed with, in addition to depression.

Not only do we expect 1 pill or 1 treatment to cure it all, we also want the results to last forever. This is unrealistic. "Cure-all" medications don't exist. Would we say the same thing about chemotherapy? "Since your cancer came back, chemo must be ineffective." Or sleeping medications ..." Since you had 2 bad night's rest while you were taking sleep meds, your medications don't work." I think we can all agree that those statements are inaccurate. I say it's a dangerous standard to set.

Just because you fall, does NOT mean you are starting over, that you are a failure, that psychedelics don't work, or that something is wrong with you. On the contrary, it means you are perfectly and imperfectly ... human. This is one of the reasons I wrote this book instead of waiting for someone "better suited" to do it. Even if there was someone else better equipped for this task with a mistake-free track record, would their message be the right one? Would a perfect experience post psychedelics set a healthy expectation for the public?

I had an early reader of *Understanding Ketamine* give me feedback — he suggested I leave the story found earlier in this book about cocaine out. "Talking about falling down the stairs after country hopping and doing illicit drugs *after* treatment doesn't really give the reader a great sense that this therapy contributes to mental wellness," he said. Well, that may be true, and I do regret that I couldn't be a better example to my readers. I understand that the topic of illegal drugs can be scary for some. Because of my upbringing, these things were much more normal to me in contrast to what I'd guess to be average. I may sound more casual than others when discussing the topic. Drugs were not scary, but rather an underlying ingredient of everyday life for my family unit. So I published this book anyway because it is important that you the reader know, not only the upside to psychedelic treatments but also the downsides, and the pitfalls to look out for.

I could have taken the reviewer's advice, left the mistakes out, and pulled the cloak over your eyes, tricking you for my own gain — this would send the wrong message, leading you to assume a cure-all approach, not to help you but to further inflate my own ego. I am not willing to do that. It is not who I am, and I will not lead you to unrealistic expectations. There are benefits to this treatment, and there are tripwires to avoid. I hope my example helps you avoid the latter. What that early reviewer was missing was simply this ... reality. Many people will benefit from psychedelics and still make mistakes, and my message is ... if it happens to you, it's ok. Get back up, like I did, and try again.

If you are reading this book, you know pain. If you don't have mental health struggles, you're reading this to get perspective on someone you love and their battles. Both roads are paved in pain. I acknowledge the vulnerability it takes to become more educated on that pain and to search for truth, knowledge, and understanding.

The toll for the information in this chapter was paid for by a pain and a darkness that I've never experienced before. That's saying a lot, considering the story of my life is similar to those described in the movies. Honestly, I never knew pain like this existed before. My life had accrued so many battle scars that I'd assumed I'd experienced the worst of it. For the hundredth time in my young life, I thought I knew, and I was wrong.

There are certain people that have good memories. They remember every detail, on every family trip, and every life experience. My oldest friend is one of those people. I, however, am not. But this year, this time, is ingrained into my brain forever. There were four things brewing that came to a head, colliding to create the deepest and darkest depression that I had ever experienced. For the purpose of this book, I'll focus on the three main sources of pain. This is, of course, speculation, because the symptoms onset was so rapid, and lasted just under a year overall. I couldn't quite put my finger on the exact source of the depression, but I have a solid idea of the accelerants.

The first was me losing my company and purpose. Second, was my best friend, more kin to a brother, evaporating off the face of the planet. The third was Covid-19 and the associated isolation, continuous governmental overreach, and detachment from relationships in my life who gobbled up their dishonest propaganda as if it were the truth.

Little by little the people I cared about were fooled, tricked and manipulated by the media. I've always had a strong internal radar for bull crap, but when I voiced it, not even my closest friends and family believed me. I had never felt more like an outsider. Feelings of isolation and anger crowded my crumbling mental state. Being alone was no longer a choice, but a requirement enforced by rules from those who didn't have my best interest at heart.

Covid-19 pandemic was raging across the world, and in the beginning, I was living in Puerto Rico. After the first case hit the island, the government thought it was a bright idea to not let anyone go outside unless it was completely necessary, like walking to the grocery store to get food. Going to the beach and exercising, for example? Forget it. Every night at 7 p.m. we were locked inside our homes. Every Sunday, nothing was open except for pharmacies.

I recall walking from one end of San Juan to the other on a Sunday at the beginning of the lockdowns. The weather was scorching hot, and I was sweating and dehydrated. I walked into one of the only stores the island allowed to be open on Sundays, a Walgreens pharmacy. I asked them if I could purchase some water. They abruptly told me no, and that the only thing they could legally sell on Sundays were prescription medications. I'd have to fix my water problem somewhere else. I mean, it made sense, right? We all know that Covid-19 was only a problem on Sunday.

When the media and government started telling us that we couldn't congregate with friends or hug family members because of social distancing, an internal alarm went off inside my body. My grandfather was in his last year of life, withering away with Alzheimer's. The family was restricted from seeing him except by appointment and in single file, never as a group. *This is wrong and I know it.* I had a serious problem with it, and the government's rules I felt forced to follow ate at my tolerance and peace of mind like cancer.

Throughout the prior years, I had been working really hard building an important business. I was stressed out. It was a supplement company to help those who'd battled with compulsive behaviors in the past, like overusing sugar, alcohol, and even narcotics. I wanted to give back to people who'd had difficulties similar to mine.

There is a predictable set of hurdles that one experiences when they stop whatever substance they are dependent on: problems sleeping, cravings, anxiety, weight gain, etc. The supplement line would tackle each one of them to give the individual a better chance at bouncing back and sustaining a new and more rewarding life, while educating on meditation and other life skills.

I had spent the previous years sharpening my e-commerce and online marketing abilities, building a team of good people in the office, and gearing up to hit the world with a product it had never seen before. The flagship supplement was named SupplementX (fictitious name).

It took me years to develop the formula for SupplementX; there were a lot of studies to comb through in order to make informed decisions with expert formulators about measurements and amounts of each ingredient. I hired the best law firm in the country in e-commerce to review my websites, terms and conditions, privacy policy, and more. I knew that the topic was a little sensitive, and I didn't want the internet marketing police to fine me down the line. "If you keep the edits we made on your pages, the risk of issues with compliance is very low," the firm said.

When we first deployed the ads on Facebook, business started booming. People were buying SupplementX left and right. I felt that I was fulfilling my purpose. I'd used my marketing and e-comm skills to build a brand that actually helped people. That was my mission: make money and make a difference at the same time.

As sales numbers grew, we gained some striking feedback on Amazon's marketplace and from emails coming in from customers. "I started drinking too much when Covid hit and this is the only thing that helped me stop the cravings," was one example. We even heard from a guy who'd recently quit using heroin while taking SupplementX, something he'd been trying to do for two years. Sixty-seven percent of customers who bought SuppementX bought it again. But I was working long and hard days, and the stress was starting to affect me physically. My neck started to clamp shut on the right side of my trap every time I sat down at the computer.

Then I received a letter from a certain government agency explaining that they had opened up an investigation against my company. It told me to freeze all documents and hire a lawyer. I was confused. I'd done everything I could to be compliant up until this point. To my knowledge, we hadn't broken any rules, and our customers loved us. The lawyers said we were good to go. What the hell, is this a joke?

The first lawyer I called to represent me said that I wouldn't get out of it without spending six figures on the defense. The accusing agency said I was violating some opiate act from 20 years back and was trying to "cure addiction." All company websites bluntly stated "this is not a cure for addiction" in three separate places on the webstore and in every footer in every landing page. Apparently that wasn't clear enough. My body was overloaded with rage, grief and stress.

The thought of losing my business, letting go of my team, and letting down my customers manifested itself in the physical world. The feeling of my life's purpose dissolving in front of my eyes blinded me with tears. By myself, on the top floor of a brick office, downtown, I started shaking and collapsed to the ground. I couldn't stop crying. I don't know what was more abrasive: the pounding of my head against the thinly carpeted concrete floor from shaking, or my heart audibly snapping into pieces.

I couldn't calm down, even as time went on. I'd read about anxiety attacks before, but it'd never happened to me. I went to the emergency room. They thought it was a joke and tossed me out the front door without any medication, help, or assistance. I'll never forget that feeling: the taste of pure powerlessness that follows the experience of needing help so badly and getting rejected.

Somehow or another, I ended up on the phone with my mom after leaving the hospital. When people talk about a mental breakdown ... I'd assume this is exactly what they are talking about. My brain felt empty and numb, like there was nothing left but sorrow. It was as if my problem solving skills, razor sharp from years of entrepreneurship, suddenly overheated. My physical body was shaking and twitching, pouring tears out of my eyes without audible noise. These weren't normal tears, but rather true pain manifesting itself in a physical form. My mother and my aunt started driving to come get me.

I'd felt depression and anxiety before, but it never interfered with my life to a point of unmanageability. There were apparently levels to this, and what I experienced that day was a much higher level. When my family pulled up to my apartment downtown, I was all but numb to the world. My tears stained my eyes and cheeks red, and my default was staring at nothing, like a robot, code written to be empty on purpose. I was indifferent to seeing my family. I knew they couldn't understand. I didn't understand, either. But I was glad to have some support and not be alone. The conversation during the drive home was anointed by awkward concern and debilitating emotional pain. It felt like hours until we got home.

When we arrived at another hospital, my mom was pretty shaken. She didn't know what was wrong with me, and I could tell that she was not only worried, but anxious about the lack of control she had over the scenario. As I was dropped off to be assessed, all I could think about was not feeling this pain anymore. "Get me something for this, please, anything," I said. I had reached my limit on pain for the day. I could no longer stand the anguish of what was going on in my brain. If anti-anxiety medications weren't made for the symptoms I was having that day, then the sky was pink and made out of leather.

The next three nights in the hospital were filled with healthy doses of Valium and antidepressants. I had taken SSRIs for anxiety before with unwanted side effects. They made me feel less anxiety, but also less excitement. I felt dumbed down, always "even" without lows and highs, like a cyborg. My sex drive was demolished, and as a young single man, that was a problem. When I tried to stop, I had brain zaps, problems sleeping, and other side effects. I didn't want to take antidepressants again. But I really needed help, so I was willing to give it a go.

Ironically, four years prior I was a pharmaceutical rep for one of the top five pharmaceutical companies in the world. My specialty was antidepressants and antipsychotics, America's most prescribed class of medications. I was very familiar with their efficacy, or lack thereof. I remembered getting trained on medications that had around a 30 percent efficacy rating, meaning 7 out of 10 people didn't get relief from taking them. Nonetheless, they received FDA approval as a depression treatment. Considering my formal education in pharma, and my own personal experiences with failing to get relief from eight other medications in the antidepressant/anti-anxiety class, my hopes weren't high. Wellbutrin, an NDRI, was the best antidepressant I'd taken in the past, so I decided to start there.

When I got out of the hospital, I was stabilized ... kind of. I wasn't sobbing and shaking anymore, but I was still very depressed. *There is no way I'd be able to function on my own like this,* I thought. So my mom and my step-dad asked me if I'd like to stay with them for a while and have some time with family. It felt like a burden, but I also didn't know what other options I had. I barely was able to peel myself off my office floor five days before, and it was a major win that I'd simply stopped crying.

My grandfather wasn't getting better. It made a lot of sense for me to stay with my family, but I feared that I'd be more of a liability than a source of help or strength.

The following half year, I was a shell of myself. I went from cranking in business to not being able to work. I couldn't even concentrate on a movie. I had completely drifted into an existence where it felt like torture just to be alive. I didn't care about the food I ate and had no energy to go to the gym. I couldn't develop relationships with my family or friends, and in public I was so anxious that I didn't know when I'd start sobbing randomly. Moping around in public wasn't a good look, and I was a liability.

In addition to the loss of purpose, a dying family member, and the government telling me I was better off sitting in isolation, the hits kept piling on. At this time in my life I had carefully crafted a small circle of friends. They were all winners. I had succeeded in surrounding myself with a solid group that constantly pressured me to reach for personal excellence and to dream bigger. My particular anchor in the group was a man named Leo. He was such a reliable friend because we had been through so much pain together. Most people who came into my life were temporary. It's how it had always been. But the test of time had hardened Leo's position in my inner circle into a rock in which I could always trust. He was a friend, and I looked to him like a brother. When he went on vacation and needed help with securing his home, he called me, and vice versa. When he had problems with his longtime girlfriend, he'd call me; and I him. Our shoulders were constantly bearing the weight of the other, back and forth and back and forth.

When Leo got smoked in his first business and went belly up, he rang. I remember giving him a free high-risk loan for $10k to start his next venture. After handing over the gold-banded green brick, I told him, "Your relationship is more important to me than money. The number-one disintegrator of strong male relationships is problems surrounding green paper; sometimes women, but as we age it's mostly money. I want you to pay me back, but if you don't then I'm willing to give this to you instead of losing you as a friend."

His eyes flashed red, then turned wet. "I'll pay you back," he promised, and he did. The reason I mention this to you is to preface the solidity of our relationship. I looked at his success as my success, and I would do anything, including losing a lot of money, to keep him as my anchor.

In the midst of all the mental turmoil I was sloshing through, Leo got into some legal trouble. In speculation, maybe his new business was so strapped he felt a lot of pressure to raise fast money to pay the bills. Either way, it was the wrong call and he was involved with the wrong people. Still to this day I have no idea what happened to him. The cartel was involved; perhaps that was part of his disappearance. I'll never know. I called and called until the number didn't work anymore. Confusion hit my cranium like a truck. Such a trusted friend, a brother, evaporated off the face of the planet, by choice. He wasn't killed, no. He chose to walk away from me at his lowest point for reasons only he and God know. I felt betrayed and angry. *How could you just up and walk away at this point in my life?* I thought. *You know I would forgive you for anything you'd done wrong. You know me, and I know you.* He knew I was vulnerable, and going through troubles of my own. Apparently, he didn't care. And it stung, from then until now; like a bee whose stinger never fell out.

This pattern continued for months. I was fighting, always in anticipation of turning the corner into positive events, but the relief never came. My doctor and I doubled down on my dose of Wellbutrin. But even months later, it made no difference. I wasn't suicidal, but after months of purposeless days and dreamless nights,

I started to think, *Is death the only way out of this? I can't exist feeling like this ... not for very long.*

After a never-ending night of emotion, my mom touched my face with both of her hands, my tears dripping onto her fingers. "You are in so much pain," she said. My eyes shut, spattering tears on the kitchen floor.

DIARY FROM KETAMINE INFUSION #10

Wherever I just went on ketamine is a place where people can vibrate and sing. That's how they communicated. I was taught about self-love and its requirement for overall health and balance. Self-care should be a higher priority.

My physical body separated from me and looped around, and I kissed myself on the lips. I laughed out loud and later asked the doctor sitting in the room if he heard me. He did. I laughed, telling him that I just kissed myself. We both laughed, again. A big statue face kissed me at the same time. It kind of looked like an ape, and he was smiling. This wasn't sexual, not at all. It was as though I could feel what they meant, as if to say, "We love you, as should you love yourself."

I saw intricate electronics, ships, and technology that looked complex.

It was dirty and the wind was constantly blowing. I was on a ship and could feel the wind when we flew in it. I could feel each time the gravity shifted under my body.

When we take off in the ship, there is a light source that moves with the propulsion and displays complex shadows like shining a light through a cage. How can this be duplicated if what I'm seeing isn't real, somewhere?

It only takes seconds to get wherever we go. None of this is cartoon-like, and it is all very realistic. I got the feeling that this reality is more real than the one I just left minutes ago. I can see, smell, hear, and feel, although I don't touch anything. This was the first time I saw humans there.

I was in a place inhabited by other people. This is the first time I've seen anything human-looking. I feel silly saying this, but I saw some beings that looked close to the aliens we see on TV. They were small and skinny, and they were operating electronics. I think they were hitching a ride on the same ship I was apparently a passenger on. They were waiting at a door of whatever I was inside of, or a portal of some kind. It's hard to put into words because I've never seen anything like it. It's all so hard to grasp.

Laughter was poured into me as if pre-loading a fountain — perhaps there's something to smile about coming up in my life.

There was a beam of light that was extremely energetic and powerful shooting into the sky. It was something so strong that touching it seemed like a death wish. I don't know what it was, but we couldn't get close to it or touch it. I think it was a beam of concentrated love because intuition told me.

You don't simply talk here, but rather feel or sing. I am very childlike in this place: curious, transparent, helpless.

Everything is so complex and yet it works so perfectly. There seems to be very little friction, very few surprises, and it seems very old. At the same time, it is advanced technologically and intricate in its archeological design.

The lesson of needing to love myself more was obvious. I retained the importance of self-care. It made sense to me. But kissing myself on the lips, I surely wouldn't have thought that myself. Who was teaching me these things, in this place?

4

WHAT IS KETAMINE AND WHAT ARE THE SIDE EFFECTS

I was afraid to even think about the fact that ketamine might not work for me. *Maybe the depression I had was too severe.* I'd heard of ketamine before, but it was mostly in the scope of people using it to get high at electronic music shows. I didn't know if it would work for depression or if it was another internet clickbait hoax designed to sell my attention to the highest bidder. I was running out of options fast. All the traditional medications were failing one by one, like dominos. With my background in pharmacology and my energy levels at empty, I reluctantly dug into the studies and research to see what useful information was available.

Let me preface my explanations by stating that because I am not a doctor or a scientist, I'm going to keep that part of the topic fairly light. If you want to know the ins and outs on the mechanisms of action, then I'd suggest reading another book. However, because of the background that I carry analyzing data, working with studies, and reading scientific literature, I'm not new to deciphering fact from fiction on the internet. I'm used to seeing how and why things work, and softening the transition from hard science to digestible info. The problem with ketamine is that it lacks strong double blind research on depression and conclusive evidence on what it's doing in the depressed brain. A large problem is the lack of proper-sized trials, often including less than 100 people. Even simple questions, like "Why does it work?" are debated. What we know so far is most people ages 18-plus seem to have dramatic reductions in depression severity when comparing traditional medications like SSRIs and benzodiazepines to ketamine treatment. The cost/benefit is favorable as well, noting ketamine carries with it a strong safety profile.

This is one of the reasons why I wrote this book: to initiate more discussion and examine real numbers on depression and anxiety treatment. What happened to me over the next year of ketamine use is not just my opinion; it is backed by a year's worth of my own data and experiences. My hope is that it all helps you understand what's possible with ketamine. Nothing in this book should take the place of medical advice from your doctor.

Ketamine is a very old drug. It was first brought into clinical practice in the 1960s and used on both humans and animals. It's touted as being one of the safest and most effective anesthetics known to medicine. Ketamine's ability to kill pain, while not depressing the respiratory system like traditional painkilling opiates do, make it a favorite tool in operating rooms across the country.

Ketamine is used to induce a state of unconscious consciousness, such as during surgery, without decreasing heart rate or impacting the patient's breathing frequency. This makes it fairly unique, as most painkillers will slow the respiratory system and decrease heart rate, mechanisms that create their own set of additional complications.

It's also considered to be dissociative and psychedelic, igniting a dreamlike state of mind in which users report seeing things in their mind's eye, and receiving insights or answers to problems they didn't previously know how to unravel. Some users report the events the ketamine unfolds as being strikingly similar to what happens to those in a near-death experience. "When I died everything went black, I saw a tunnel ... there was a light at the end of the tunnel" ... you've heard the stories before. During the four surgeries on my arm and hand after breaking my back, I was given ketamine through my IV each time.

Under proper medical applications, ketamine is generally considered to be very safe, but just like any drug, there are always downsides to consider. The side effects of ketamine are dose and frequency dependent. One group of researchers found that ketamine was harmful to the bladder lining, causing "ketamine-induced cystitis." It is not common unless one abuses the medication. The condition is triggered by inflammation and causes ulcers in the bladder lining, so it is perhaps the most alarming side effect to discuss with a provider if undergoing treatment.

Side effects are often present when ketamine is abused, and include memory loss and reality dissociation. The list of common side effects from normal patients who aren't abusing the drug are mild, for most but can include anxiety, increased heart rate and blood pressure, dizziness, and muscle tension.

ABUSE POTENTIAL: This is important to consider when weighing the positives and negatives of any drug, even those prescribed. Ketamine has a moderate potential for abuse, not because it feels all that great in comparison to other drugs, but rather because it can reliably and effectively change the way you feel. So, surprise, people like to get high on stuff. Based on my experience with the drug and the research that I've done, abusing ketamine can cause problems — just like taking too much Tylenol can cause liver damage and death. If you don't do it alone and work with your doctor, the odds are strong you'll be just fine.

Starting in the 1980s and continuing throughout the electronic music scene, ketamine made its way into the pockets of concertgoers and psychonauts eager to explore the edges of human consciousness. It adopted a popular term, not to be confused with the popular cereal, "Special K." Traditionally, users take veterinary liquid ketamine vials, empty their contents on baking sheets to dry in an oven, then scrape up the white crystalline powder, piling it into colorful baggies ready for use or resale.

Ketamine is used as a tranquilizer of sorts, and that's the best way to describe what happens to someone when they recreationally use it. Depending on the dose, users report extreme relaxation and vivid dreamlike visions. If pushed too far, then one may fall into a "k-hole," which is the term used to describe what it feels like to be "stuck" on ketamine. In this state, the user finds themselves unable to move, and the body and consciousness they know so well dissolves into a zillion pieces, to the point where they pretty much cease to exist on this planet.

I've never had a good experience using ketamine as a recreational drug. Until the present point in my life, I'd tried it two or three times. Once, I accidentally slipped into a k-hole, and each time I felt uncomfortable and had a hard time moving my limbs. It's an unpleasant experience to maintain consciousness while blind and paralyzed.

In South America, a new drug based on ketamine was recently born. In Medellin, Colombia, the cartels introduced a pink or purple powder that included a mysterious set of ingredients unknown to users. No one really knows what's in it, and that's part of the sales pitch. One time, I had a guy offer to sell me the formula when I was eating lunch. "It's called "Tuci" (Too-see)", he said. "And the formula is a secret. I'll sell it to you for $6,000."

It was bright pink, with flavoring complete to make it smell good when being sniffed. I don't know what is in Tuci, exactly. In general, no retail buyers do, hence the price tag on the formula. I can speculate, though. One thing I know for sure is ketamine is the most prominent ingredient in the mix.

MDMA, caffeine, methamphetamine, and sometimes even fentanyl complete the ever changing party-time cocktail ingredients list. Go to a club in Colombia. The pink powder you see on everyone's nose is not cocaine, it's Tuci. Some people claim to be physically addicted to it. Ketamine can have withdrawal symptoms when abused, so that doesn't' shock me. And fentanyl and meth, if included, are among the most addictive substances on the planet. But the mixture feels good, so young people are willing to gamble with the cocktail, even though they don't know the ingredients. I've stayed away from Tuci, myself. Variables can be dangerous and negatively affect emotional stability, depending on what substances are mixed in the ingredients for the day.

On the other hand, it is hard to abuse ketamine when strictly using it medically once per month via infusion. Sniffing a bag of Tuci in a South American dance club is a different story.

Since the drug is reliable in doing the same thing each time, it is easier to abuse. People who abuse drugs are trying to escape the way they currently feel. When making the choice of which substance to use, the more predictably effective, the better. This is why alcohol addiction is so rampant. It works really well every single time. You don't have to worry about becoming mind-numbingly paranoid or seeing eyeball-eating dragons on alcohol. Ketamine is like the alcohol of the psychoactive class, it's predictable but abusable.

5

A DRAMATIC HISTORY

Ketamine's evolutionary impact on mental health started to steal the focus in 2006, specifically in the area of treatment-resistant depression. But there was one major problem: the drug is old and its patents are long gone. In the pharmaceutical business, drug companies usually earn a patent with a drug that grants them the ability to sell it for a certain period of years. Right now, that period is 20 years. This means the manufacturer of the drug has sole rights for the duration of their patent, and nobody else can sell it or make generics for two decades. When the patent expires, other companies are allowed an expedited approval process to make generics, and in most cases, clinically equivalent versions of the original drug.

This change in the monopoly structure of the initial patent period disrupts the incentive for the first mover. Now the price of the drug is all that matters, and it's a race to the bottom: whoever can make it the cheapest wins. Profits are drastically reduced, and the upside of patent protection is gone. There are companies that thrive in the generics business, but as a general rule of thumb, if a drug can't be patented then businesses won't pursue it. When businesses don't pursue it, research and funding evaporates with it.

In 2012, off-labeled ketamine clinics for depression and chronic pain treatment started to catch fire, and by 2019, the FDA approved an altered version of ketamine called "esketamine." Up until this point, ketamine was traditionally given as an "infusion," a procedure in which a doctor or anesthesiologist administers a steady dose of ketamine over a period of 40-60 minutes as the patient sits in a recliner with headphones and eye shades on.

This new molecule of ketamine is different in two ways. First, it has a different delivery method and is given intranasally, as a nasal spray. And two, it's a small alteration in the original ketamine chemical. The alteration maintains ketamine's efficacious mental health properties, but changes it enough so it receives another set of patent-protected years of profitability.

Alterations like these represent a pretty common practice. If something can be altered, changed, or isolated in a medicine that works well enough to get a new patent, then oftentimes companies will allocate resources to making the monopoly game come to life. I'm not saying this is what happened here, but based on my knowledge of the business, it's a common practice and makes perfect sense in a capitalist medical system.

Esketamine is delivered as a nasal spray and not intravenously like traditional ketamine. Therefore, it has a lower bioavailability than the traditional drug. Bioavailability refers to the amount of drug that is absorbed into a person's bloodstream. The traditional route of IV ketamine is around 100 percent, and esketamine's nasal application comes in at approximately 48 percent. The benefit of esketamine is that it was approved by the FDA as a mental health treatment, so insurance companies often reimburse patients using esketamine for depression. Since traditional ketamine mental health treatment is "off label" at the time of this writing, getting insurance to cover it is like playing the lottery ... odds are really bad.

When I was making the decision on whether or not to pay the $400-$500 per infusion of traditional ketamine, or to try and get insurance to cover esketamine, I landed on paying out of pocket for the real thing. I made phone calls to providers, both of esketamine and ketamine, and the response was across the board more positive for the traditional medication. The data that I gathered online showed that IV ketamine is 70-83 percent effective in treating treatment-resistant depression, and esketamine is about 40 percent. Intravenous ketamine seems to be significantly more effective, but in time brings more statistically significant numbers. With twice the bioavailability, it makes sense that the original would likely work well. Considering the only data that I have to present in this book is from the traditional IV ketamine infusion practice, that version of the medication will be the focus in the chapters to come.

6

HOW DOES IT WORK

Let's consider for a moment the touted efficacy (effectiveness) and information available on ketamine in regards to depression. Warning: this chapter is a little medical and technical. If ketamine research doesn't interest you, skip this chapter by just knowing the following: ketamine does need more research in the mental health space. A lot of the studies on how it works were done on animals. Without large human studies on depression, it's challenging to talk about numbers. The studies we do have suggest ketamine does work, rapidly decreasing depression symptoms. But how it works is another story. If you don't care about research on how ketamine works and why it's effective, then you can move on from this chapter; I don't want to lose you. If you do care, then read on to learn what I mean.

When I stated that the reported success rate of ketamine in reducing depression score is 70-83 percent, my first reaction was "I doubt it." One of the main reasons is this: we aren't talking about patients with depression. We are talking about treatment-resistant depression, a condition including only the orphan people who don't respond to traditional medications used in this class (Celexa, Zoloft, Prozac, etc.). For a percentage of people in our society, these traditional medications are enough. But what about the others — the treatment-resistant depression crowd left behind? Nothing is working in the traditional Western medicine arsenal, and you're telling me ketamine carries a reported 80 percent success rate for THOSE PEOPLE (like me)?

To put it mildly, it was a lofty claim. Considering other FDA-approved medications skate by with efficacy rates under 50 percent for normal, non-treatment-resistant people, an 80 percent success rate for the depression orphans is almost laughable. If this is true, then what are we doing over here messing with inferior medications, decade after decade after decade, suicide after suicide?

It made no sense to me, frankly, and was so outlandishly unrealistic I immediately discredited the statistic.

I dug in further to poke holes in the claims. I wanted to know how and why ketamine seemed to work so well for depression. The infusions were very expensive, and a pain in the ass to execute. I'd have to get a ride to and from the doctor's office after each infusion. I'd have a set of six infusions back to back over a period of two to three weeks, and then one every three to five weeks after that. Just like taking an antidepressant, maintenance was required. Instead of taking a pill every day, I'd be signing up for an infusion once per month. Although it was better than having to take a pill every day, it was a big ask. I'd need to be convinced.

One thing was clear: there were thousands of people and physicians touting ketamine's praises and saying it worked on the internet, but where was the significant science? Perhaps the most telling of studies I read was said to be "a substantial breakthrough" in how scientists understood how ketamine affects the brain circuits. Until this point, they had strikingly little understanding as to what might be going on under the hood, despite the positive results seen at the infusion clinics.

Previous research found evidence to support the fact that ketamine creates new "synapses," the connective matter between brain cells. But this new study seemed to answer questions about how and when the new synapses actually affect brain function. However, there was one notable hurdle — the study was on mice. "There's probably no such thing as a depressed mouse," said Dr. Conor Liston, a neuroscientist and psychiatrist at Weill Cornell Medicine in New York. Dr. Liston was the author of the scientific journal on mouse study. But the silver lining was mice do feel the effects of stress. And luckily for Dr. Liston, stress mimics depression.

Liston and his team of scientists in the US and Japan gave the mice a stress hormone designed to make them act depressed. Sure enough, they lost interest in their favorite activities like exploring their maze. They even lost interest in eating sugary foods. "Stress is associated with a loss of synapses in this region of the brain that we think is important in depression," Liston says.

Consequently, the synapses started dropping as their stress levels increased. Liston started giving the mice ketamine while measuring synapse growth and development. Within a very short period of time — sometimes within minutes — the mice started to regrow the same exact synapses, in the same configurations from before the stress was introduced into their diet. It seemed to support the theory which claims ketamine may restore the parts of the brain that were damaged by stress, in less than six hours.

The study didn't explain why ketamine was repairing the brain so fast, but it did explain why ketamine may work to relieve depression in people. In less than six hours, the brain connectivity was functioning better, and the mice as a whole stopped acting depressed. But, "It wasn't until 12 hours after ketamine treatment that we really saw a big increase in the formation of new connections between neurons," Liston says.

The conclusion was drawn that ketamine may work in a two-step process. First, it may help faulty connections with stress-related damage function better temporarily, and afterwards restore synaptic connections altogether for a longer-term fix.

What was interesting about my findings was there were both physical and metaphysical reasons for why ketamine could potentially work for me. The two-step process outlined above was the physical. If ketamine did, in fact, start repairing damaged cells within minutes, and continue to support new connections in the brain, then it would make sense that positive changes in mood could be possible. But what about the visions on ketamine? What were the benefits to those?

I'd argue the drug does not have a two-step process, but a four-step process. One to two are assumed in the above study, and three to four I derived from my own personal experiences. In step three, a user deciphers the teachings and communication that one has with God (or

The Universe, The Higher Self, or whatever word you want to use to describe the lessons taught to you in the ketamine world). Step four, a user integrates and applies the relevant knowledge into their life.

7

WHAT ABOUT THE OTHERS

My ketamine research and experience is strikingly similar to other psychedelics. For someone who has had all the mental health problems in the world, my battles have forced me into the boundaries of medicine and back. I am not provided the luxury of taking big pharma's word for it, shutting up, and not asking questions.

It seems like the West, as developed as we are, is so blind to anything outside the box. We take it to the point of denial, limiting the scope of what is possible or appropriate for the suffering individual. If you've suffered like I've suffered, you know the feeling ... when everyone tells you to do this or that, and NOTHING works.

Or when the doctor barges in the room, talks for five minutes, gives a diagnosis and a pill with a host of side effects, and then doesn't see you for another month or three to see if anything has actually improved. It's a terrible feeling. I'm not a quitter, so what options does one have when the media and professional treatments fail, if not to give up? The option is to search and to learn, and throughout the years I'm grateful that's what I've chosen.

The history of this drug class is filled with drama. One major problem with psychedelic compounds is that many of them grow naturally. Even more, there are different types of psychoactive plants growing in every region of the world. In areas like Antarctica, where plants can't grow as easily, you'll find psychedelic mammals. With 200 different species of hallucinogenic mushrooms alone, it's almost like Mother Nature is making a point of their importance. What are all of these things doing here, naturally growing, not only intertwined but essential to our ecosystem?

Ketamine and LSD, for example, were both thought to be manmade — until recently. Ketamine was newly found as a natural occurrence in fungus. What we thought was a pure synthetic is actually a naturally occurring psychedelic, although ketamine does differ from others in the natural psychoactive class. We can assume, however, that the synthetic version of the drug will continue in favor because it's easier to produce consistently. Natural or not, the similarities in the visions and messages received are undeniably coincidental. The messages of the importance of love, interconnectedness, and compassion for oneself and others are common. These themes have duplicated across species and survived for centuries alongside the timeline of human evolution.

There are many examples of psychedelics both natural and otherwise, but many of them differ in how they interact in the brain. Some of them have a dramatic effect on serotonin, have a high affinity to the receptor, and are called *serotonergic psychedelics.* These include LSD, psilocybin (Mushrooms), DMT (Ayahuasca), and Mescaline (Peyote Cactus). Some prefer to describe them using the more formal term, *tryptamines.* Ketamine is different, primarily interacting with the NMDA receptor.

LSD was first synthesized in 1938 by a man named Albert Hofmann, and became known as a cure-all for hard-to-treat mental illnesses like alcoholism and depression. Research was booming and the results were nothing short of mind-blowing. LSD had essentially changed the game of psychiatry. It was common practice to have guided LSD sessions with a therapist, and it was working for the vast majority of people.

One of those people was Bill Wilson, the founder of the most successful substance abuse treatment group in history, Alcoholics Anonymous. Bill and his wife gave credit to LSD for curing his depression. Bill was also attempting to quit smoking. From what I've gathered, Bill was taking acid with his therapist for numerous years, beginning in 1956. During this time, Bill was updating AA literature and speaking across the country. The third edition to Alcoholics Anonymous's Big Book was completed almost 20 years later, in 1976, five years after his death. When someone is new to AA, it is generally recommended they read two books, the "Big Book" and the "Twelve and Twelve." These two books cover the group's approach to recovery in detail, as well as outlining the 12 steps and 12 traditions that make up AA.

Letters to and from Bill's therapist, his wife, and to other members of AA suggest that Bill was taking LSD and/or mescaline while writing and developing the format and later literature of Alcoholics Anonymous. Bill's results with LSD were so profound he approached the original members of AA with an idea. He believed a spiritual experience, a belief in a higher power, was required to stay sober. But there was a problem ... some people just didn't seem to receive that connection. They would stay sober for a couple years, and then they'd relapse. The one common denominator was a lack of spiritual connection.

Bill suggested that AA members who had trouble finding a higher power be allowed to use LSD to find that connection. Based on his experiences in guided LSD therapy himself, including group therapy with his wife, he was convinced that this could solve the issue. The hierarchy of AA denied him, and he developed a reputation of sorts with the more conservative members. To this day, most AA groups will tell you taking a psychedelic like mushrooms or LSD is considered a "relapse." But according to the founder of the program itself, it may be quite literally the opposite.

Part of the speed bumps developed along the evolution of psychedelics started in the late '60s and early '70s with the rise of the anti-war movement and hippie-fueled flower power. LSD had crept outside of the therapist's office and was being used in ways that were not just endangering people, but the governmental and media structure itself.

The famous story everyone hears about is someone jumping off of a building to their death, thinking they could fly because they had taken LSD. I don't know if that ever happened or not, but I've heard it plenty from the generation before me. People were abusing it, and people were defying the powers that be and protesting against the Vietnam War. War is big business. This became a problem.

Despite the promising wave of groundbreaking mental health treatments throughout the '50s and '60s, psychedelic medicine and psychoactive plants were criminalized in 1968. From the natural psychedelic fungi to the lab-made LSD, the whole lot was placed into the Schedule 1 narcotic class. There are five numerical values for drug classes, Schedule 1 being the most harmful, Schedule 5 being the least. In order for a drug to qualify for a Schedule 1 placement, it must meet certain requirements.

The definition of Schedule 1 goes something like this: a drug or other substance that has a high chance of being abused or causing addiction and has no medical use in the United States. All the data and scientific research up until this point on psychedelics was shoved into the denial pile and ignored for reasons only God knows. To give you an idea of the hypocrisy here, crystal methamphetamine is a Schedule 2; that means it has a lower potential for abuse and has more medical value. We have no data showing psychedelics are addictive — in fact, quite the opposite. The visions and experiences ignited can be scary and unpredictable. Imagine 20 years of therapy jammed into a four-hour mushroom journey. It's not exactly the best recreational drug, considering the other options, and it's certainly not addictive like methamphetamine or predictably pleasurable like cocaine and painkillers.

Throughout my early life experiences in recovery, I have never met someone in a treatment center, self-help group, AA meeting, or rehab that was addicted to psychedelics. Not one. But I've known countless that have died from seizures induced by alcohol addiction. America's drug of choice is tremendously toxic if abused. In my experience, psychedelics done in the wrong setting, like in big groups or at parties, can be scary and cause paranoia. This is why I never touched a psychedelic from the later stages of high school until the age of 30. All of this was rumbling around in my brain as I considered the option of ketamine therapy to treat my depression. I had to weigh the cost against the benefits, and the 70-80 percent-plus success rate seemed incredibly high and was hard to believe.

8

WHAT MAKES KETAMINE DIFFERENT

There are many similarities and differences between substances in the psychedelic class. The species of plants dot the entire world and span from corner to corner of the map. The synthetics, like ketamine and LSD, are made in a lab. The naturally occurring ketamine found in fungus is relatively new, so for the purpose of this book, we'll keep that as it is. Any psilocybin (mushroom's psychoactive compound) taken in the West for research or legitimate medical use, at this time of writing, is done via a synthetic version as well.

There are two types of science in the world. One type of science is safe, predictable, accepted, and researched in prestigious universities around the world. This type of science studies things we already know to be true, like gravity or the ability to treat disease. The other science pushes the boundaries of what humankind knows to be true. It crawls the edges of human awareness, pushing the limits and boundaries of all we've come to know and accept. This is where space exploration comes in, and this is where psychedelics are today.

Fast forward ten years, and I can see researchers isolating all of the useful psychoactive chemicals in every plant that has a medical benefit. It makes them easier to distribute around the world, and allows the doses to be easily controlled. When doses are easily controlled, there is a measure of predictability introduced into a notoriously unpredictable medication class. Following that standard is a measure of safety. I think this is a good thing.

The similarities between plants and synthetics alike are very interesting. The science shows us that ketamine acts completely differently than other serotonergic psychedelics. It is, however, similar in its ability to impact to the default mode network in the brain. The default mode network is where we store the memories or stories of who we are.

> ***Definition 1:*** *The default mode network (DMN) is a network of interacting brain regions that is active when a person is not focused on the outside world.*

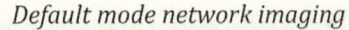
— sciencedirect.com

Default mode network imaging

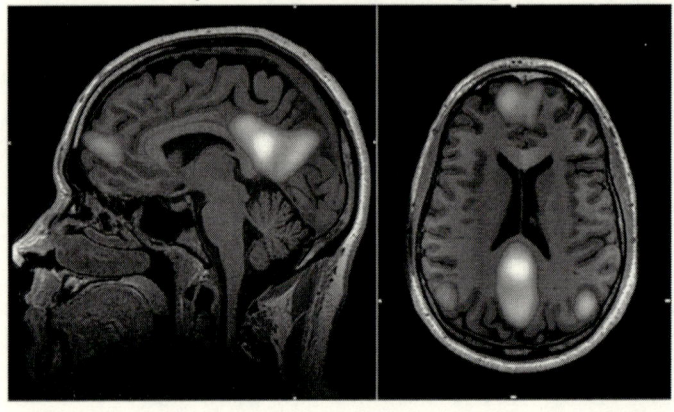

Definition 2: *The default mode network is active during passive rest and mind-wandering, which usually involves thinking about others, thinking about one's self, remembering the past, and envisioning the future rather than the task being performed.*

— wikipedia.org

Wikipedia nailed it this time. In simple words, this is the part of the brain that gives us feedback on what should and shouldn't be. It tells us how poor we are and how ugly we are. The monkey on our shoulder, or the devil, its impact depends on the significance of negativity that it chirps. Either way, it's annoying.

This part of the brain is automatically running at all times when we aren't focused on one specific task, and can be active even then. The DMN is less active in those who have a meditation practice. Seasoned practitioners are said to have lower baseline DMN activity. This is the part of the brain where the ego lives, or our ideas of self and how we fit into the world around us. The ego is what keeps our identity protected, and is shielded from change by the veracity of the individual's DMN.

When most think of "ego," they assume confidence. It can be quite the opposite. The ego is the construct of one's self which puts pressure on the individual to display confidence, or whatever best matches the ego's definition. When the ego construct is inflated, so too are the expectations of one's self; spilling over into often inflammatory behavior. A bigger ego brings with it a louder devil, whispering in our ear, "You're a screw-up."

When those around us report back about experiences in meditation and psychedelics alike, they bring with them similar tales. They tell about out-of-body experiences, and a striking understanding that what was being witnessed is, in fact, rooted in a rather obvious but unseen truth. LSD, mushrooms, ayahuasca, ibogaine, peyote, and ketamine all teach the same messages. The locations the user is sent to and the experience itself vary dramatically, but the lessons are always the same.

Reminders of the importance of love and compassion for oneself are common, along with an interconnectedness to the universe, plants, and all living things. Users find a sense of "oneness" with God, learning lessons of what is truly important in life, and are able to solve problems that were otherwise impossible to see clearly. People report reliving traumas of the past and forgiving themselves and others for wrong actions. The science of psychedelics is now measuring the severity of the "mystical experience" through a series of questions. Like tests, these questions are scored and added up to measure the severity of mystical experience revealed to the patient. The relevance is striking. The more powerful the mystical experience, the more lasting and sticky the positive outcome becomes.

I should add, negative trips are possible and they can be scary. Most of this can be avoided with proper screening of patients because psychedelics are not for everyone. Tremendous care should be taken in the setting in which these drugs are explored. I've been blessed to be able to afford to work with doctors and shamans in South America and Mexico, always giving respect to the local tradition of medicine ingested. That should be the desired route because the farther we stray from caution, the more likely negative things are to happen. Scary things do arise.

When I was in Peru, three of the eight-person class left after night one because it was too intense for them. One girl had a bad reaction and ended up in the hospital. Others just got freaked out after watching idiotic videos on YouTube about ayahuasca, without properly understanding the severity of the mission they were embarking on. I prepaid for a week of ayahuasca ceremonies and got so rattled on night two I never did it again. These substances are not a game. Those trying to make small changes in their life probably won't have the desperation needed to take the risk of the traditional four-to-six-hour-long vision quest that feels like twenty years of psychotherapy. Ketamine, although more controllable and predictable than other psychedelics, can cause feelings of anxiety and loss of control.

"Set and setting" is also incredibly important. What is the mind state of the individual undertaking psychedelic therapy? Do they have underlying conditions? What is the environment like and is it safe? Psychedelics like ketamine can exacerbate schizophrenia, bipolar, and other personality disorders. When I started ketamine infusions, I was broken and desperate, so I took the risk; in every other instance of psychedelic use, I have been very particular and careful about my present mind state. These substances have a tendency to let you know when you're ready. If you don't feel ready, don't do them. This is where the lines of use and abuse are drawn. Most of these substances are really hard to abuse because of the significance and unpredictability of experiences.

This is where ketamine is different from other psychedelics. It is the most abused out of them all, and I have a few thoughts as to why. The ketamine experience, although extremely diverse in lessons taught and visions seen, is relatively predictable and stable. The infusions last around an hour and are controlled by a doctor, giving flexibility of dosing in real time. When patients have a bad experience on ketamine, the doctor can cut the medication and administer another medication to help the patient calm down in a matter of minutes.

These are benefits unseen in other psychedelic practices. If you have a bad or hard trip on ayahuasca, you have no choice but to hang on tight and see where it takes you. This is not always a bad thing; users report the most healing following the hardest experiences.

Ketamine is predictable and calm, lowering the volume of the DMN lower and lower until it's quiet and as thin as vapor. The DMN volume reduction experienced on ketamine is dose dependent and can vary from person to person. Generally speaking, it is a dependable and stable drug that works very effectively every time it's used, and this is why it's abused significantly more than the other psychedelics.

Fewer bad trips are reported during ketamine infusions because of the mildness of the experience in comparison to ayahuasca or mushrooms. The latter species can completely shatter reality for hours and hours at a time, while ketamine is more gentle and shorter. I always knew who I was, where I was, and what I was doing while undertaking ketamine infusions with my doctor.

The experiences on ketamine are a bit harder to retain and integrate into life. This is another important difference to understand which will further strengthen the reality of expectations. As you may notice, I had to immediately diary the experiences I had on ketamine, or else they would fade quickly in time. I'm not sure what the reason for this is, and if I were to define it, it would be speculatory. Although the experiences were often very meaningful at the time, their memory and significance seemed to leak like sand sifting through an hourglass. Eventually, there is no sand left. Other, more intense substances present an experience more akin to undergoing a savage-like spiritual battle and coming out of the other side victorious. These experiences are often more meaningful, and therefore easier to retain, then integrate into life.

9

LIFT OFF

Very little of what I'd worked on to improve mental health when I was younger had worked for me. Therapy, self-help books, 12 steps, doctors, institutions, and so on, were never internalized into processes I could actionably carry out in my life. They never helped me accept myself for who I am. When I say I've retained a little from the traditional treatment routes, I mean close to zero. The exception is AA (Alcoholics Anonymous), which taught me the power of being vulnerable and is probably partially to credit for me displaying my naked heart for you to see in these pages. Prior to ketamine, my first true experience with psychedelics happened by accident at the age of 30. I was confused but very intrigued, and it opened the door to considering ketamine to treat my depression.

My first psychedelic experience in Thailand severely impacted my life. I will tell you this story in my next book. The experience had faded in time, however — not leaving, but becoming more fragile in its ability to prop me up. As the days past the memories floated farther and farther away. The deep, depressive symptoms didn't start to accumulate for years after Thailand. I cry every single time I write about it because whatever happened to me there meant so much. But this depression situation was a different beast altogether.

It didn't seem to matter that I knew I was loved, and worth more diamonds than there are sand; if there was no direction or conduit to channel that love, it didn't matter.

What if ketamine really could repair depression-related damage in the brain, had a 70 percent-plus success rate on the hard-to-treat cases failed by traditional medicines, and could induce mystical experiences like I had that night in Thailand? Sign me up and let's go. I had nothing left to lose besides my life. I hadn't quite reached the cliff of suicidality, but thoughts about ending my life to relieve the pain I was feeling inched me closer to the ledge. It was only a matter of time, I think. To this day, I wonder how long I could have lasted.

The misery of me not being able to be me was the darkest reality I had ever seen. I had suffered for so long. I didn't have much tolerance for it anymore, or maybe a better word is endurance. It had been almost a year straight of strangling depression and stress. I couldn't function in life. Emotionally and physically, I was drained empty.

In the following two chapters, you'll find a compelling case to support treating anxiety and depression by using ketamine via infusion. This dramatic data set stretches twelve months and eighteen visits long. Every appointment started with me answering around twenty check-in questions on two tests. These were measuring grids which allowed the doctor to decode the severity of my depression and anxiety symptoms since my last visit.

All the scores and data gathered from my physicians are 100 percent real, and the impact was made of something so special I can't tell you too much about it until later in the next chapter. Whenever in doubt, it's usually best to let math and numbers do the talking. Honestly, I don't get too excited with math, but I've been forced to study statistics in the e-commerce business. Don't let the numbers lose you. I promise, they are easy to understand. And what I've found is, unlike humans, numbers don't lie.

My first infusion was booked after a mental health provider referred me to the ketamine clinic. It was now years ago, in December. When you're too sick to function day to day, the memories blur and bleed together until the days and moments become hard to recall. But I remember being excited by the potential of help, and I kept a diary to record what I felt and saw. There was a doctor there, and a nurse or medical assistant of some kind. First they asked me to fill out the two tests to gauge my initial anxiety and depression scores. They are standard tests in the United States, and are called the GAD-7 and PHQ-9.

The PHQ-9 (see example below) is a nine-question test with five tiers of depression severity. I went through the questions and tallied my rankings. When you receive a depression diagnosis, this is how they measure the severity. My score of 22 landed me at the top of the five tiers, "Severe."

The GAD-7 (see example below) is a different test with four tiers of anxiety levels. My score of 18 also landed me in the "Severe" category. I was still taking Wellbutrin, terrified of what I'd feel like if I stopped. But the scores reflected confirmed that it was not working and I needed more help. My depression scores were so high that they recommended to the doctor I'd likely need a higher level of care (i.e., hospitalization of some kind) if the treatment did not work. Below are the PHQ-9 and GAD-7 scores from my second infusion. The first was worse but wasn't accessible at the time of writing.

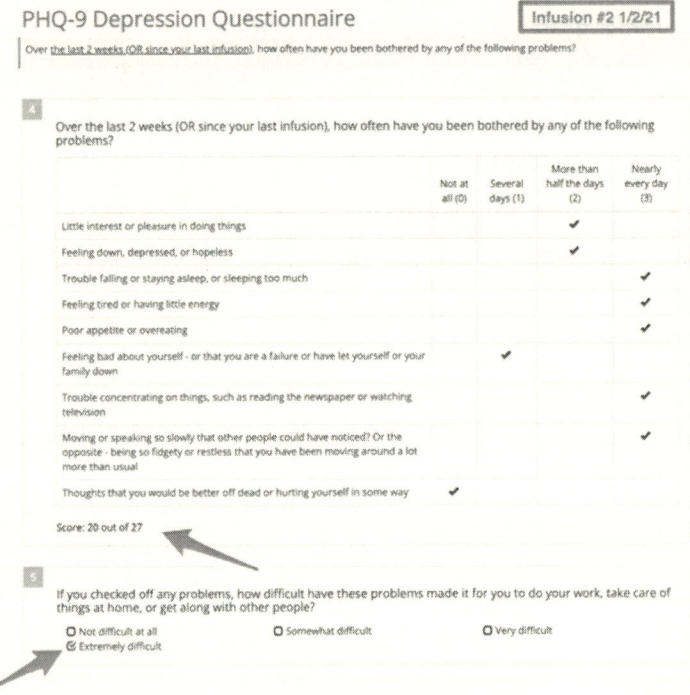

PHQ-9 from my second visit

Treatment considerations based on score: (2)

Proposed Treatment Action by PHQ 9 Score

PHQ-9 Score	Depression Severity	Proposed Treatment Actions
0-4	Non – Minimal	None
5-9	Mild	Watchful waiting; repeat PHQ 9 at follow-up
10-14	Moderate	Review treatment plan if not improving in past 4 weeks; Consider discussion of additional support such as pharmacotherapy
15-19	Moderately Severe	Consider adjusting treatment plan and/or frequency of sessions; Discuss additional supports such as pharmacotherapy; For SonderMind Anytime Messaging clients, consider converting from asynchronous to synchronous therapy channels
20-27	Severe	Adjust treatment plan; focused assessment of safety plan and pharmacotherapy evaluation/ re-evaluation; If emergent then refer to higher level of care; Likely Not a candidate for asynchronous/text therapy

PHQ-9 rating system

GAD-7 Anxiety Questionnaire

Infusion #2 1/2/21

Over the last 2 weeks, how often have you been bothered by the following problems?

1.
Over the last 2 weeks, how often have you been bothered by the following problems?

	Not at all (0)	Several days (1)	More than half the days (2)	Nearly every day (3)
Feeling nervous, anxious or on edge				✓
Not being able to stop or control worrying		✓		
Worrying too much about different things				✓
Trouble relaxing				✓
Being so restless that it is hard to sit still				✓
Becoming easily annoyed or irritable			✓	
Feeling afraid as if something awful might happen	✓			

Score: 16 out of 21

2.
If you checked off any problems, how difficult have these problems made it for you to do your work, take care of things at home, or get along with other people?

☐ Not difficult at all   ☐ Somewhat difficult   ☑ Very difficult
☐ Extremely difficult

My GAD-7 from my second visit

Treatment considerations based on score: (1)

Score	Risk Level	Intervention
0-4	No to Low Risk	None
5-9	Mild	Provide general feedback, repeat GAD-7 at follow up, consider adjusting treatment plan if not improving in last 4 weeks
10-14	Moderate	Further evaluation recommended; For active treatment plans consider adjustment; For text therapy clients monitor for synchronous therapy
15+	Severe	Adjust treatment plan; focused assessment of safety plan and pharmacotherapy evaluation/ re-evaluation; If emergent need then consider referral to higher level of care; Client is not a good candidate for text therapy/asynchronous

GAD-7 rating system

As you can see from the above examples, I wasn't feeling well. Even with infusion number two in the above illustrations showing 10 percent better scores than infusion number one, I was still "severe" in both categories.

10

WHAT DOES A KETAMINE INFUSION FEEL LIKE

When I arrived at the ketamine clinic, the doctor instructed me to sit in the back of his office, in a 12x12 room. It was large enough for a big recliner, a desk with a computer, and room to navigate the IVs and medical equipment. Trying to gain my confidence, the doctor told me that if things got weird during the infusion, or I got anxious, he could give me a variety of medications to calm me down. They hooked up an IV in my left hand, and gave me a puffy set of headphones with a preloaded list of songs specifically constructed for ketamine infusion therapy. I brought in eye shades to cover my eyes but would still be able to open them.

I wasn't prepared for what I was about to experience because before my first infusion, I didn't know the psychedelic effect was so strong in ketamine. I thought the visions produced on mushrooms and others were surely more pronounced because I hadn't heard about people's personal experiences on ketamine before. And although the psychoactive experience is milder than others, the visions were as clear as looking through a windowpane without glass. The ketamine experience was similar to what people see with a near-death experience. That's all I knew about the ketamine realm. Calming, right? At the risk of sounding silly or new age, I'll do my best as a writer to describe what happened to me there. I'll let you decide for yourself what it could mean.

INFUSIONS:

When the medicine went into my body, it was slow and controlled. The first thing I noticed was the volume of the voice on my shoulder started to dim; the default mode network, mentioned in chapter 8. If you've had a meditation practice before, it's a similar feeling. You experience less negative feedback, magnifying the present moment. For me, it's a place that is a lot quieter.

The beginning of the infusion felt like slipping into deep meditation. This is the initial phase of quieting the DMN.

As the medicine ramped its way up, and my eyes were closed, I started to see a white dot bouncing around blackness. A really weird thing about ketamine is that it never mattered if my eyes were open or closed; I'd see the same thing either way. It's kind of like a dream, but one you are conscious and aware of. I knew I was in the office and getting treatment with a doctor. I was aware of my surroundings, observing this mysterious dot bouncing around the black canvas of my peripheral. My physical body started to stiffen and become rigid, almost as if that was part of the process of leaving it. It felt like I was a snake leaving its body, preparing for something new by shedding old skin.

As the dot got closer, the visions began, cloaking my whole mind in the walls of a tunnel. Mimicking the same reports by those who've come close to death. I was moving through a malleable tunnel made of what seemed to be a vaporous material. I felt calm and was not nervous. The music was soft and calming, and it seemed to guide me into a dreamy state effortlessly. It's difficult to explain what happens at the end of the tunnel.

Somewhere between the process of dimming the chatterbox brain volume in the DMN and moving through this tunnel, I felt like my consciousness had left my body. I knew where I physically was, but my awareness dropped into a room at the end of the tunnel. Every infusion, every time, I went through this tunnel and landed in the same place. It looked like a tomb, with stone walls and earth's crust as a ceiling. It was always stormy there, the wind constantly kicking up dust and scattering rocks along stone-speckled paths.

The colors there were darker and included lots of gray, greens, and browns. The texture of the walls, buildings, and natural landscape were clearly marked, as if I was now sitting in a new place quite similar to Earth. I'll probably never forget what the stars look like in this place. There were thousands of them everywhere, scattered across the sky and bright as ever.

I saw technological hubs nested into the sides of rocky cliffs, illuminated by colored green, purple, or blue fluorescent lighting tubes. Because the place was so dark, there were often lights illuminating whatever needed to be. The lights were intriguing. I would often get a panoramic view of my surroundings, like the panning of the camera in *The Matrix*. These fluorescent tubes would illuminate the tech hubs, casting shadows and changing as the light source adjusted to the panning movement of my view. The shadows would dance, always intricate and obedient to the moving shadows cast by each separate light source. Rules of reflection identical to those we all know.

My infusion experiences were always pretty similar in physical location, but never duplicated in visions or lessons. One aspect that was always exactly the same, however, was the importance of love and purity. I would find myself in front of large carved rock statues, and what seemed to be gatekeepers of sorts. They'd move in front of me and radiate this energy in my direction, communicating the importance of who they were, or what they represented. It was always love that they cared about, and they seemed to want to measure if I had the capacity to share mine. They were obviously important, and had been around for a long time. They reminded me of what would be found in a well-preserved archeological dig.

During each infusion, after floating around in the rooms at the end of the tunnel, they'd scan me for the presence of love and who I was as a person. It was almost like they wouldn't let me in unless I was some sort of good guy with positive intentions. Sticking my chest forward, I'd do my best to communicate who I was without speaking or being spoken to. In the beginning infusions, I remember trying to communicate to them, "Please, let me in. I need help. I am really sick." After scanning me for 10 to 15 seconds, the statues always let me pass.

I was always shown a lot of grace here. Without the comfort of my ego or physical body, I felt vulnerable. But

I was never exploited or scared or hurt. It was almost like those things didn't even exist. Unlike other psychedelics like mushrooms or ayahuasca, there were never any dark or scary experiences here. Never. Traditional psychedelics always have a dark door that can be opened or stumbled through, but that is not my experience with ketamine. Bodiless, and with my heart as my only compass, I'd float around from vision to vision.

I was never in control of anything. I was always the observer, but always being observed. Something was running the show because the trip was linear. It would start in one area of my life, or one hurdle, and the visions would build on themselves like a movie, only to circle around at the end for closing credits on introspection. Each vision was masterfully crafted and woven into an intricate puzzle of meaning. Sometimes I'd be placed on spaceships and moving from one location to the next — yes, I'm a smart guy, and I understand how crazy that sounds. But nonetheless, if you're this far in, I'll just tell you ... I don't know what it all means, but these are things I saw.

I was often being rocketed silently from place to place; it was like traveling by warp speed in the movies, when the stars stretch linear and it only takes five seconds to get there. What is that? It was always one of my favorite parts because my body would actually shift with the gravitational pull of what I was experiencing in this other place. If we took off in a ship, my head would be thrown back physically in the doctor's office. If we tilted or turned during a vision, my body weight would reflect the intensity of the movement. I often experience things that my mind fails to make sense of, no matter how many options I run through. *How is it possible for my body to shift in the real world based on things that my consciousness is seeing in the ketamine world?* I wondered. I'll likely never know.

The mysteries presented here seemed to increase the effectiveness of the therapy by stretching the limits of everything I believed to be true. Limiting beliefs began to crack. The best way I can explain it is that each infusion felt like a tune-up. And each time my outer shell would soften a little more. Each doctor's appointment morphed into a reminder of what is important in life.

Predictably and continuously, I'd bring my worldly stressors into a session, then interact with them in a space where I could actually see them for what they were. It was kind of like wiping raindrops off your glasses; it's easier to see. Oftentimes, the takeaways were simple and easy to digest, like: "You have a purpose. You can't stop now because I chose you." Sometimes they were difficult, like when my grandfather died and I saw him in a vision. He was happy, and he wasn't sick anymore.

It's hard to explain the healing that takes place in interactions like that — seeing the dead, and all. I was sitting in front of my recently deceased grandfather, tears streaming down and seeping out of my eye shades. He didn't say a word, rolled up right in front of me in his wheelchair, and smiled. That's it. It meant so much to me to see him, and it gave me peace seeing him happy.

The vastness of the variables experienced in this place is hard to put into words. The technological advancement was made of something from the movies, and since I didn't recognize it, I can't say what it was. There were people there, pilots that occupied the cockpits of ships. Animals sometimes embodied a conscious human or operated machinery or electronic items. Wires were running everywhere and into everything, powering this strange world and illuminating the darkness. A striking blend of mysterious tech and archaeological history enveloped my consciousness, though each time I returned to the same exact place.

THE MOST IMPACTFUL EXPERIENCE I HAD ON KETAMINE

In my next book, I'll teach you everything I know about ibogaine, an African psychedelic plant whose roots, when ingested, send users on a vision quest and simultaneously reboot the opioid receptors in the brain. I want to stick to the topic at hand here, ketamine. My experience with ibogaine and ketamine collided on the last infusion with my first ketamine provider. During this intersection of psychoactive approaches, I had the most powerful infusion experience to date. Please keep in mind, using two different chemicals back to back can have negative consequences, so consult a provider as I did.

I had just returned from Cancun. Ibogaine is illegal in the West except for Mexico. It is also commonly used in Costa Rica. My experience was so meaningful and powerful that I couldn't sleep for one week afterwards. I didn't care. The gifts I'd received during the process outweighed the negatives. I felt so lucky to be able to see what I saw. To feel what I felt was a privilege that most can't afford. It was $10,000 to go. The only reason I was able to was because of the flexibility of my schedule and financial stability. Ten days after returning from Mexico, I was cloaked in gratitude. My mom commented at the time, "Something is definitely different about you." The experience changed my perspective dramatically, and I felt so lucky.

To this day, I'll never know what caused such a dramatic shift in my ketamine experience. I have a feeling the variable was gratitude and humility. It wasn't often that I carried these traits into my ketamine infusions. Usually by the time I went to my infusions, I was slightly off track and needed a kick in the ass. This was different. I went into my ketamine infusion so grateful and humbled to have experienced powerful lessons in Mexico. But everything else, like ketamine dosage, time interval between visits, etc., was unchanged.

Usually, I'd end an infusion with feelings of gratitude and humility. It wasn't until the last infusion that I started with them.

DIARY: 12/30

The usual flight through the tunnel, the transfer to another world, happened as usual. But this time, I didn't stop in one place. I had a feeling in my chest, similar to a "gut feeling," showcasing the level of humility and gratitude I was entering with that was propelling me to new levels of awareness. It felt like I was emotionally leveling up, and I was finally starting to develop spiritually. Whoever was controlling the ride was rewarding my gratitude, recognizing it as I was propelled into new levels of development. It felt like I was emotionally leveling up.

I kept going to new levels, boom, boom, and BOOM! I finally ended up in space, somewhere in the sky, with a downward view of planets and stars. From right to left, all I could see were bright twinkling stars, and placed in between were soft silhouettes of planets.

It seemed like a perspective only God would be allotted. I instantly felt guilty and that I wasn't worthy of such treatment. All I could see was the sky, and it was clear that I'd never been this far out before. I was told, "Don't you see? You are still learning. This is what you have to look forward to if you stay on this path." I was told that Jesus was God in human form, which is odd, considering I haven't claimed Christianity since I was a child.

I wouldn't find out until later that many people come to organized religions through psychedelic compounds. Similar to AA's founder Bill Wilson and his LSD endorsement, It's just not talked about openly.

I was brought down out of the sky and back to the ground. There was a presence here that felt like the same one that was talking to me in the sky. As I got closer, I could feel it — stronger and stronger until I couldn't stand it any longer. I crumpled into a pile on the ground under the weight of this power. I felt the most concentrated energy source I'd ever felt before in this place. It was so strong that I couldn't stand with the weight of it pressing me down like gravity. I thought that God or Jesus could pop their head around the corner and walk up to me at any second.

As I sat in a heap on the ground, it kept telling me, *"You are the one. All of your pain is for a purpose. I am molding you. You were chosen by me."* I kept saying in response, "No, not me. It can't be me. I'm just an imperfect man, it can't be me. Please, don't choose me." As I write this, I get emotional, remembering the lack of judgment and the faith that this power had in me.

When I said this, I started absorbing all the energy out of the things around me. The trees, rocks, and ground were feeding me with an energy of some kind, helping to power me up with confidence. Things that I couldn't see but only felt were doing the same. It violently kept pouring into me until I started to become more powerful myself.

With the help of this unseen force, I started to gain confidence. Self-doubt and fear began to leave me. I started to cry from a feeling of intense gratitude. My cheeks and eye mask were drenched in tears.

I ripped my face mask off, turned to the doctor, and said, "Did you feel that?" He said, "Nope, everything was normal on this side." I sat there with my head in my hands, crying, not able to move because of the shock radiating through my cranium.

"That was God. My pain is for a purpose. I am chosen to do something important," I thought.

I didn't move or speak for ten minutes. The doctor observed me and sat silently. The silence was broken with the only words that could possibly begin to explain what had just happened to me. "I think I just experienced God," I said to him.

11

THE RESULTS

Time after time, each session chipped away at my symptoms, and the numbers gathered were powerful. I can go on and on about different things that I saw and did, but what matters most in this story is what happened and how it worked. This is where we bring the physical (science) into the metaphysical (non-physical), and bridge the divide with easy numbers. Remember the GAD-7 and PHQ-9 tests for anxiety and depression? When I started ketamine therapy, I was ranked as severe on both, pinning the top of all symptomatic categories except being suicidal.

Within ten days and four sessions, my symptoms started evaporating one by one until my scores reached those of a normal person. My PHQ-9 (depression) plummeted to a 3 from a twenty-two, and my GAD-7 (anxiety) dropped from eighteen to five. They stayed that way for the whole year. All the while, my dose was not increased. Take a look at the images below to see what I mean.

My PHQ-9 and GAD-7 scores for the year

```
1. Score, Doses, Meds
       12.       : PHQ9: 3, GAD7: 5. Dose given: 0.86mg/kg (70mg, 81.7kg), zofran 4mg IV
1 Yr   11.       : PHQ9: 6, GAD7: 2. Dose given: 0.86mg/kg (70mg, 81.7kg), zofran 4mg IV
       10.       : PHQ9: 2, GAD7: 6. Dose given: 0.86mg/kg (70mg, 81.7kg), zofran 4mg IV
       09.       : PHQ9: 3, GAD7: 4. Dose given: 0.83mg/kg (70mg, 84kg), zofran 4mg IV
       .         : PHQ9: 2, GAD7: 2. Dose given: 0.83mg/kg (70mg, 84kg), zofran 4mg IV
       07.       : PHQ9: 1, GAD7: 7. Dose given: 0.83mg/kg (70mg, 84kg), zofran 4mg IV
       06.       : PHQ9: 9, GAD7: 8. Dose given: 0.81mg/kg (70mg, 85.5kg), zofran 4mg IV
       05.       : PHQ9: 2, GAD7: 4. Dose given: 0.81mg/kg (70mg, 85.5kg), zofran 4mg IV
       04.       : PHQ9: 2, GAD7: 4. Dose given: 0.81mg/kg (70mg, 85.5kg), zofran 4mg IV
       04.       : PHQ9: 4, GAD7: 7. Dose given: 0.81mg/kg (70mg, 85.5kg), zofran 4mg IV
       03.       : PHQ9: 9, GAD7: 9. Dose given: 0.81mg/kg (70mg, 85.5kg), zofran 4mg IV
       02.       : PHQ9: 9, GAD7: 8. Dose given: 0.81mg/kg (70mg, 85.5kg), zofran 4mg IV
       02.       : PHQ9: 6, GAD7: 5. Dose given: 0.81mg/kg (70mg, 85.5kg), zofran 4mg IV
Day    01.       : PHQ9: 6, GAD7: 5. Dose given: 0.81mg/kg (70mg, 85.5kg), zofran 4mg IV
10     01.       : PHQ9: 3, GAD7: 5. Dose given: 0.81mg/kg (70mg, 85.5kg), zofran 4mg IV
       01.       : PHQ9: 5, GAD7: 5. Dose given: 0.81mg/kg (70mg, 85.5kg), zofran 4mg IV
       01.       : PHQ9: 15, GAD7 12. Dose given: 0.81mg/kg (70mg, 85.5kg), zofran 4mg IV
       01.       : PHQ9: 20, GAD7: 16. Dose given: 0.7mg/kg (60mg, 85.5kg), zofran 4mg IV
Start  12.       : PHQ9: 22, GAD7: 18. Dose given: 0.58mg/kg (50mg, 85.5kg), zofran 4mg IV
```
Severe GAD7 and PHQ9 scores turned normal in ten days.

I find this quite interesting because of the delicacy of the topic. It's my desire to display facts. And this topic is as fragile as it is mysterious. I don't want to tell you about everything I saw while trying to grasp at an understanding that I'll likely never reach. I don't understand where I went on ketamine. I want to see real-life impact. I'm after the results. I don't like to take stories and fairy tales and attach them to factual statements. I believe in data, and I believe the efficacious nature of this medicine is twofold. For me, there was a physical reprieve of symptoms almost instantaneously. Secondly, the visions and lessons gave me the fuel and hope needed to make changes within my day-to-day life. The visions gave me courage; not from what I saw, but rather what I felt.

Do not miss this. My PHQ-9 and GAD-7 tests were taken 18 times over the course of 12 months of infusions. I'll repeat: I went from severe depression and anxiety to a normal human in 10 days. I continued to bounce around the bottom of the charts for the entire year. I ranged and bounced back and forth from normal to mild, never to return to severe again.

PHQ9 Scores and Proposed Treatment Actions		
PHQ9 Score	**Depression Severity**	**Proposed Treatment Actions**
0 to 4	None	None
5 to 9	Mild	Watchful waiting; repeat PHQ9 at follow-up
10 to 14	Moderate	Treatment plan; consider counseling and/or therapy
15 to 19	Moderately Severe	Active treatment with medication and/or therapy
20 to 27	Severe	Medication treatment and if member shows severe impairment and poor response to therapy, refer to mental health specialist for psychotherapy and/or collaborative management

PHQ-9 from severe to none/mild in 10 days

Proposed Action by GAD 7 Score

Score	Risk Level	Intervention
0-4	No to Low Risk	None
5-9	Mild	Provide general feedback, repeat GAD-7 at follow up, consider providing your patient with behavioral health resources.
10-14	Moderate	Further evaluation recommended; provide your patient with SonderMind resources.
15+	Severe	Provide with SonderMind resources. Assess safety plan and pharmacotherapy evaluation; If emergent need then consider referral to higher level of care.

GAD-7 from severe to none/mild in 10 days

DIARY 1/7

This is the first time I went into an infusion feeling good, and not down or crappy. I was told I was chosen again ... I'm reminded of this almost every time. It's as if it's telling me to keep going, keep pressing forward. I'm supposed to do something.

It's kind of scary working on myself here, without the ego whispering in my ear. But I like the real me. I'm very childlike, curious, loving, and emotional.

I saw tremendous visions the whole time. I was told that I was "almost ready" for something. I can only assume that it is referring to moving out and buying my own house (which I did months after), or being ready to date again.

I was told that money is mere rocket fuel to expose people for who they truly are, and I haven't been the best example, myself. If someone is cocky, money will make it worse. Money is an accelerant to an individual's character traits.

It's bizarre that the physical world reacts to what I'm seeing and doing here. For example:

- *I can feel the wind when flying*
- *I can feel gravity when falling*
- *I can smell what it smells like there*
- *I can feel the temperature drop and have often needed a blanket because it's so cold*

I have a powerful heart to love and this is where the fuel for life exists. The nucleus of our being is perfect and so beautiful. This life is not what we think it is. It's some sort of training ground.

I hope I can use this knowledge to live more carefree, be patient with myself, and just have fun. I want to be more lighthearted. There's no reason for me to be so anxious and worried all the time.

At one point, I felt totally exposed in my body, but no matter how vulnerable I feel, I still feel like I'm going to be okay. I'm able to fully trust. I'm able to stand tall, and just be me. Communication is different there. Feeling is how communication is accomplished, not words.

It's hard to describe, but everything revolves around love. Love seems to be the fuel that everything uses to function well. It seems to be the interconnectedness between everything. In its absence, nothing works properly.

Back in my body, I feel pretty out of it. The crazy thing is, it doesn't matter if my eyes are closed or open; I see the same thing. I tested this out multiple times and when I shut my eyes, it's the same. How is that possible?

When my doctor sent me the scores in preparation for this book, I couldn't believe it even though I'd lived it. After every medication failed, just under one year of agony, and POOF — like that, my depression symptoms were all but gone. They had evaporated; never to be felt in totality again. I remember at least three times when I came out of an infusion in tears; I told the staff, "Thank you so much for helping me. I don't know if you realize how important your job is here. I think you are saving my life."

Since starting the ketamine infusions, I was able to come off of my antidepressant medications and I never started them again. The ketamine worked so well at alleviating my symptoms that one day I just didn't have to take them anymore (please be cautious when discontinuing medications, as many SSRIs have withdrawal symptoms).

I've had three doctor-prescribed ketamine sessions since, but never felt I critically needed them. The desperation of that time of my life has left. When I got hurt and broke my back, I was prescribed so many narcotics during the recovery process that my doctor had to take me off of ketamine. He didn't think it was safe to continue treatment with all the medication I was on. I was worried my depression symptoms would come back without taking ketamine. That never happened.

My life isn't perfect, and anxiety is still a default of mine, amplified by stress and dependent on the day. But the darkness of the well of depression is a depth that has never returned to me. I don't know if I'd be alive or dead without ketamine. That's the truth.

Every time I got picked up after an infusion, riding through downtown Seattle, I saw tents stuck in neat lines side by side, down and across all sidewalks. My heart would sink deeper into my chest. The only variable that separated me from those people was that I had money and resources. I could afford it. People need help today more than ever. They deserve options and education despite their level of income.

I have a strong feeling that psychedelic therapy will continue to evolve slowly, with rich people benefiting first and poor people last. This is unfortunate, and should be solved by the entrepreneurial community as fast as humanly possible. It's my hope that I can do a little to help that happen with this text. Education is an inexpensive format.

I want to accelerate responsible and safe treatment by exposing what these substances are, what benefits and negatives they carry, and what my experiences with each of them are, as a patient in controlled settings. This book is part of the mission, but I have a lot more to tell you about in my next release. I have already paved the way in pain, so there is nothing left to do but share my experience and knowledge.

12

INTEGRATION

The problem I see with ketamine is that it works really well for many people — too well. I never confirmed the 70 percent-plus metric from my initial research was, in fact, true. Statistics are often easy to swing. Considering the dramatic decrease in my own symptoms, I am no longer so skeptical and have opened up to the possibility of such efficacy. It worked so well for me, and so rapidly, I had a hard time balancing such a dramatic change in my life. Without continued work and self-care, psychedelic therapy via ketamine treatment will likely fizzle out, the significance fading alongside time. Emotional maintenance is a necessity if integration into life is expected. I didn't do the best job at this.

While sitting in the hospital bed with that big brace around my neck, and my arm ripped to shreds, I thought, How am I going to get out of this? After all I just went through with depression, and now this. I wasn't prepared for the battle with pain medication lining the horizon. It had been too long, and the desperate memories of my difficult past had faded with a decade's time. The infusions worked so well that I had become lazy and overconfident in my ability to manage extreme difficulty. Asking for help is problematic for me. At that vulnerable point in time, which I will tell you about in my next book, I really should have.

Psychedelics treatments are relatively new, and the integration step is underdeveloped. As a consequence, I have admittedly been a bit of a lab rat. There was no paved road for me or proven systems to follow. Family and friends alike expressed concern toward my "different" approach. But they haven't walked in shoes like us. Soles worn from the failures of modern medicine. It was a risk I was willing to take, considering the consequences of doing nothing were undeniably large. The significance of my turnaround is tainted with mistakes. I'm confident that if I had a proven system of aftercare to step into, there would have been less of them.

My first ketamine provider offered services with one man. He was a psychedelic therapist, which means he helps people decipher the significance of their experiences and integrate the changes into their own lives. He charged $200 per hour and didn't take insurance. This was and is an unfortunate reality of where we sit. I never met with him, although he sounded quite busy. There are not many good resources for psychedelic therapy yet, and aftercare is definitely one of the shortcomings.

What do I mean by aftercare and integration? It can be working with a therapist weekly to discuss how treatment is going and how to apply it. Attending therapy is positive because it can provide a layer of safety when "life" happens. Life always happens. The question is, how prepared are you? I was not very prepared, and I attribute that to overconfidence, ego, stubbornness, and most of all lack of options.

Aftercare and integration can be working with a group of likeminded people in a similar structure to twelve-step groups. AA is not successful because of its treatment plan to get people sober — they don't even have one. The group is successful because of its focus on providing a community for the individual after they escape their dependency and start life again. It works because there is work, accountability, vulnerability, honesty, companionship, and likeminded struggle. According to a well known psychedelic treatment coordinator practicing in Mexico, patients have a better chance making changes that stick when constructing an aftercare plan including counseling and group therapy.

Until someone builds an aftercare and integration structure into psychedelic medicine, people will continue to fall through the cracks. In the meantime, the job is ours. Responsibility for integrating these powerful experiences is fleeting, and setting up our own self-care is required if the expectation is to sustain better results.

For me, psychedelic therapy has been like playing bumper bowling. As I zigzag through life, these compounds have allowed me the ability to stay relatively in-bounds. When and if I step outside of bounds, it feels so uncomfortable and so unlike me that I can't wait to get out and pull the e-brake. Scratching and clawing, I always pull myself out. It didn't used to be that simple.

What if we didn't need to fight so hard and had other options to make the lessons experienced on psychedelics stick more effectively? I have gathered ten ideas to support psychedelic integration and lasting change based on my own experiences, with the continuous cycle of trauma and failure as my witness. It is overwhelming to expect perfection in them all. These are mere ideas and are not meant to be rules, just as they aren't to be done all at once, by everyone. Take what you like, and leave the rest. I am not attempting to be the psychedelic poster child. I hope it helps.

 Scan the QR code to have the following ten integration techniques delivered to your phone so you can customize and make them your own, it's free.

1: PRAY

Having a relationship with a higher power is a practice humans have engaged in since the dawn of time. Today is just a glimpse of history. We have enormous religious structures that illuminate individual paths to what I choose to believe is likely the same destination. When taking psychedelics, restricted ideas about God and its existence are oftentimes shattered, and at the very least are bent permanently. It's my experience that becoming closer to God is a daunting task, and the resolution isn't always obvious.

The pressure these medicines put on the ideology of God's non-existence is so great that integrating a small amount of prayer is a logical next step with very low risk. A relationship with a higher power can be helpful, but the word "relationship" also implies work, communication, listening, trust, etc. It's a two-way street in every example I can name, so why would it be different here? Not knowing exactly who I'm praying to is much less important than the act of praying itself. Sometimes I get on my knees. This is something I learned in the last infusion that I described earlier. Stepping into the metaphysical, into prayer, with humility, is likely a powerful place to be.

2: SUPPORT SYSTEM

I hate this word. I've heard it a million times. "Mr. Daniel, you need a support system." Unfortunately for me, it's true. Fortunately for you, I have gone before and made the mistakes, so technically you don't have to. If you're anything like me, however, it may take your own mistakes to actually learn from them. A support system is loosely defined as people you can talk to candidly about experiences, shortcomings and battles, and get advice from. It can be friends from a self-help group, people from church, colleagues at work, or a variety of them all.

I am very deliberate about who I bring into my circle of support. I look for people who have something that I want. It could be expertise in a topic, rigorous honesty, or the ease in which they seem to navigate life. This now provides fertile ground for an environment of learning and growth. Most importantly, the number-one ingredient required in this support system is diligent honesty. If I can't be honest with someone, and they can't be honest with me, then I cannot rely on them for support in this area of my life.

3: THERAPY

Therapists have haunted the dreams of Americans for decades. God knows they haunted mine for many years. It's not fun opening up to someone, especially when the life story told is one of constant horrors. "Where do you want me to start?" I'd ask whenever a new therapist requested my story for the first time.

Therapy provides an interesting combination of benefits, which is why it's included in this list of ten integration techniques. Therapists are trained listeners, and even if not in psychedelic medicines themselves, are usually quite open to listening to the experience and providing feedback. Using them as a sounding board helps them understand what you've experienced and may give them insight into ways to turn an experience into integrated actions. They also can provide a ripcord for uncomfortable life events. Stuff happens; it always does. Having someone there to listen has been more positive for me than negative. If the counselor relationship doesn't fit, I move on to the next one until it does.

4: MUSIC

Integration is about maintaining emotional stability. Music is a fantastic way to massage buried emotion; especially when creating it. Is there an instrument you want to pick back up again? Is there something new you want to learn? Do it.

One of the largest goals of psychedelic integration is to remember the profoundness of the experience. The senses of smell, sight, and hearing are among the best tools we have for intricate recall of the past. If we do not anchor the experience with something useful, it is easier for it to slip from memory. When undergoing modern-day psychedelic treatment, it's always accompanied by music. Request the playlist from your provider. Listen to your favorite songs, especially the ones you remember playing alongside your most dramatic victories and lessons. This practice has helped me remember the things I never want to forget.

5: DIARY, THEN READ THE DIARY

Keeping a diary of the psychedelic experience is crucial. This practice has served the contents of this book in a few ways, the most obvious being the ability to recall and relive events that were positively and negatively impactful during the experience. Keeping the diary contents fresh is another matter. I've found that reminding myself of what happened in days past on psychedelics can be beneficial to my current day. There are a variety of ways to remember it. One of them is reading the contents of the diary. I've read them quite often in preparation for this book. It made me realize how much I forgot, and revived lessons that had faded into distant memory.

6: EXERCISE

This one is a bit macro. Exercise has little directly to do with integration, but everything to do with mental health sustainability. Where do most screw it up? They skip the days they don't feel like going. The best businesspeople, the best athletes, don't only show up when they feel like it. The best show up when they don't feel like it.

I'm not saying that we need to become pro athletes here. But I do think the unsustainability that haunts most workouts is simply being too comfortable and wanting results easily. I'm having a day like that right now as I write. I don't want to go to the gym today, and I'm tired. What I do in this case is just do cardio. I still show up, and I grind it out on the stair stepper. Boom, done. Mental health box checked.

7: MEDITATION

I can see your eyes rolling from here, and that's okay — I get it. Mediation is not easy, it's hard. It takes practice, which is why they call it "practicing meditation." The science of meditation revealed earlier in this book says we can quiet our monkey mind permanently with a meditation practice. If you are like me, and the monkey in your mind is loud, then this may be a ticket out. A breathing technique I like is this:

Sit in a chair or on a pillow with your back straight.

Breathe 5 to ten full breaths using the belly to expand the lungs, instead of the chest.

Breathe in through your nose and out through your mouth.

On the next breath, take in as much air as you can possibly take in, then at the top of the breath sip in a little more.

At the top of the breath, with full lungs, wait for 5 to ten seconds.

While you wait, clench and hold a root lock (which basically means, clench your butthole).

You may feel pressure in your head.

After 5 to ten seconds of holding, release your breath out the mouth and nose simultaneously, letting go of all tension.

Sit at the bottom of the breath for 5 seconds, then repeat the large deep breath 2 to 3 times before returning to the normal breaths.

8: BREATH-WORK

There are classes for breath-work that teach breathing techniques which also impact DMN activity; they help you experience an awareness similar to psychedelics but without the drugs. This age-old practice has been used to heal the mind for centuries. I found this to be an amazing and peculiar resource that can be useful when trying to get in touch with emotions and deep-seated traumas. I used to go to breath-work class every week. It would often make me cry. One example of breath-work is listed above, in #7 Meditation. If you are curious about more, Google "breath-work classes" in your local area. It is not easy to execute on your own because your body will constantly tell you to stop. But if you have the fortitude and willingness to push through those thoughts, you will be dramatically rewarded. Breath-work also dims the DMN just like psychedelics. It sounds crazy, and silly. But I promise you, if you execute the following, it will surprise you. Here is a breath-work technique I was taught and have used recently with staggering mental benefits.

Put on some soft music that provokes emotion. The breathing over the next 25 minutes should strictly be from your mouth. Never mind all the negatives you've read about mouth breathing. That suggestion is primarily during movement. You'll be just fine.

Lie on the ground. Breathwork can cause your arms and legs to go numb and feel wobbly. Don't try to get up until you're ready.

Take a big breath into your belly, then another into your chest. Let out the breaths in the same sequence through your mouth and relax. Into your belly - Into your chest - Out and relax. In - In - out. Repeat this pattern for 25 minutes straight. Do not quit and stay the course.

The hardest part is getting through the first three songs. If you can make it that far, then you're almost home.

Thank me later.

9: TAKE OWNERSHIP OF YOUR MISTAKES — PAST AND PRESENT

"Keep your side of the street clean." You might have heard that before. This should probably be number one because it is so critical. Being honest and owning up to actions that are negative provides an amount of breathing room unrivaled by mere silence. There is something special about keeping your chin high and an internal peace that comes with knowing you're doing the best you can, and when not, promptly acknowledging it. This is something directly out of twelve-step self-development programs.

I also encourage ownership of mistakes in the past. Apologizing is critical, especially when something comes up in the experiences to show you how you're wrong. It is very common for psychedelics to illuminate dark corners often ignored in normal states of consciousness. My actions are a product of my thinking, and taking ownership of wrongs helps fortify to yourself and the other person the fact that "they are important." The negative thing about apologizing is that they can't constantly be rapid-fired out. If the apologizer is always executing the same infraction, then what's the point of the 10th apology? The apology is worth more when the apologizer is in a good place in life, where the receiver can have some trust or reassurance that you actually mean what you say.

10: BUY SOMETHING THAT'S A REMINDER OF THE SIGNIFICANCE OF THE EXPERIENCE

During one of my most meaningful visions, I had in my company a bodyguard of sorts who sat behind my right shoulder. He was dark-skinned, from Africa, and only had one eye. His head was large and round; he reminded me of Mike Tyson. One unlucky eye socket looked as though its eyeball was plucked out in a knife fight. I stared wonderingly into his skull.

"You don't gotta' worry about nothin. I got you. To the motherfuckin bone!" he growled repeatedly so I wouldn't be scared of the things I was envisioning.

I bought a statue for the front of my house that reminded me of him to keep the memory fresh and the experience significant with time. Now I'm reminded of each lesson learned every time I see him at my front door.

Even with the dramatics of my turn-around on ketamine, I still have life obstacles to overcome. My depression has evaporated like rain on a steaming blacktop, but the trials will never end. This is the nature of evolution and the subsequent nature of fear. I am sure now all struggles are for a reason. I believe that God tests its strongest soldiers hardest to prepare us to fight for purpose. As you will see in my next book, the slippery slope created by the confidence instilled by these medicines is a force within itself.

These medicines are incredibly effective at interrupting negative thought patterns and providing a window of reflection. Most people are given a period of time with increased clarity to execute changes in their lives. But they are not a cure, and change requires action. To complete a lifelong positive upgrade, it often requires more than just a pattern interrupt to be holistic. Change is only as sticky as one's effort behind it. It kind of reminds me of when I became financially free. It's one thing to make money, but keeping money requires a completely different set of skills. And developing those skills, like anything, requires action.

13

THINGS TO CONSIDER BEFORE GETTING A KETAMINE INFUSION

If you are seriously considering ketamine infusions, this last chapter is for you. This class of medication is strong and tends to have a mind of its own. There are a few preparations that can increase the probability of a more controlled and beneficial experience. In ketamine's case, since the medicine is slowly entering the body through an IV, the doctor can manipulate the experience in various ways. This is a benefit to ketamine, but it is still not to be underestimated. Here are a few things to consider when searching for a provider and starting therapy.

Music plays an important role in our mood. Think about gym music versus wedding music. This variable can work in your favor or against you. I have learned to take the advice of the provider and use their playlist, assuming they have successfully treated patients before you. These playlists introduce songs made to impact your mood, in a therapeutic way. Different frequencies are used on purpose to guide the experience into positive and emotional places. Hard rock or techno, for instance, is probably not the best choice for working through trauma.

Music choice can be fairly obvious. However, I've had two providers, one of whom did not have a specific playlist. I'd consider this a red flag and if I was a new patient, I'd find another provider who has one prepared. If this is not an option, there are playlists on Spotify that I'd recommend. (Scan the QR code to visit the resources page to download.) Always remember to switch your phone onto airplane mode or do not disturb. When deeply sedated, it's quite distracting and confusing to get alerts.

Choosing a provider can be a bit overwhelming. Here are some things to consider. There are different use cases for ketamine with different protocols and doses. For instance, chronic pain treatment uses much higher doses of ketamine administered through a longer period of time. This is not the focus of this book. An infusion itself should run 45 to 60 minutes and include time for recovering. After the treatment you will be disoriented. My body felt like a robot afterwards, and it's hard to walk for 10 to 15 minutes. All providers in my city at the time of writing charge $400-600 per infusion, with the average clinic charging $500. In preparation for this book, I called all of them to relay the information to you. The variation in price can be a variety of things, like the amount of staff present in the room, or the number of patients being treated at once, or the "environment experience" in the office. From a patient's perspective, here's what's important:

- Does the doctor treat more than one patient at a time? If they do, does a nurse stay in the room with you at all times? I've experienced both; the first clinic's doctor stayed in the room during the infusion, the second did not — and neither did a nurse. There should be a nurse and a doctor at minimum in the clinic, and in my opinion, one in the room with you at all times. Here's why; when you wake up from an infusion it can be quite confusing and scary if you're in a room by yourself. The opposite is true with a professional in the room. Sometimes you may have questions, or feel uncomfortable, or need someone to talk to. You will not be able to walk, so if you're stuck in a room on your own it can increase the chances of experiencing anxiety or fear, and if you get up and try to call for someone it could be quite dangerous. This is why the protocols being developed for psilocybin (magic mushrooms) treatment recommend two people in the room at all times during psychedelic therapy.

- What type of device do they use to administer ketamine? There are different types of ways to administer the medication via an IV. The first and most controlled is using a timed plunger/syringe which administers the medication based on a time interval. This is my preferred method, as it seems to provide a more controlled entry point into the experience, with a gradual decline. The other method includes a timer attached to the IV that releases the solution into the body using gravity. I've used both, and the latter is more violent in its entry and exit from the body. I'm not exactly sure why that is, but I can speculate that the weight of the solution in the bag changes as the volume of liquid is reduced throughout the session, so perhaps the change in volume has an effect on the weight and therefore an effect on the rate in which the medicine is delivered. Again, this is speculation. The positive to this device versus the large timed syringe is that it makes no beeping sound when it's finished. Some people may get startled by the audible alert. If you've had surgery, you may remember waking up to a loud beeping sound that alerts the doctor when the timed syringe is done administering the anesthetic.

- Do ketamine providers require a pre-authorization from a mental health provider? Ketamine providers themselves are doctors, but they are usually anesthesiologists. They are not psychiatrists. Most clinics will require the green light from your mental health provider acknowledging you are in fact "treatment resistant," have tried other medications and failed, and are medically encouraged to engage in ketamine therapy. It's a pain in the butt, but it's a sign that they care. Some of these doctors don't care and are just in it for the money. I've found, the further you can get away from those types of providers, the better. Comfortability and safety is the goal. And this is one way to check.

- Another way to vet providers is to check if they monitor PHQ-9 and GAD-7 scores. Every appointment should start with two tests measuring your anxiety and depression symptoms. If the provider doesn't monitor this data, then how can they decide on dosing or know if the treatment is working? If the clinic doesn't monitor your scores, find one that does. At the very least, be monitoring it with your mental health physician.

- If you'd like help selecting a pre-vetted ketamine provider in your area at no cost, refer to the "resources" page at the end of the book.

Transportation is a big concern. If you thought you'd be driving to and from the infusion appointments, you're mistaken. After the infusion, it will be impossible to drive in the first couple hours, and it is encouraged not to drive for a full 24. This means the clinic will require you to schedule transportation to and from your visits. Some clinics allow Uber, and some don't. Check with insurance to see if they offer transportation services to appointments that require anesthesia. Most clinics prefer a friend or family member to be in charge of transporting you.

Things to bring with you. During the infusion there are a few necessities to bring.

- Eye shades, or a "sleeping mask" are not only necessary, but they vary in effectiveness. You want one that does not let any light inside, zero. It should not wear easily, change shape, or warp over time. These masks (scan the QR code to refer to the "resources") are the best I've found because they don't let any light in, are rigid, and allow space for you to open your eyes while wearing them. Traditional masks, like the ones assigned on an overnight flight, scratch my eyes if I open them. It's a high probability that you will cry during treatment. Masks with sponge material along your cheeks help to wick moisture.

- Warm, comfortable clothes. The more comfortable you are the less likely you'll need to communicate or adjust something during the infusion. Avoiding changes midway through is helpful because it's difficult to move during treatment. I found a blanket helpful, and always kept one within reach.

- Bring your own headphones if you are worried about sharing. Some clinics have in-house headphones and others do not. Heads up!

*Write in an integrative journal. I like to set an intention or goal for the infusion. Write it down. Example: I want to release my anger towards XYZ or I need help loving myself. This is common practice in psychedelic treatment around the world. Do not let unanswered intentions deter you. If your request is not answered, ask again. I also find a journal helpful to write down the things I learned and saw which I want to integrate into my own life. Say you learn the importance of self-love. Write down what you saw and how it made you feel. Then jot down a couple ideas on how you can practice the lesson. Example: Start yoga classes again or Don't look at my phone or emails first thing in the morning. Put it away until 10 a.m.

What medications are you taking? This is a big one, and if you've vetted a provider properly then they should have addressed this with you already. You should know, there are medications that diminish the effectiveness of ketamine treatment. When I broke my back and had all those surgeries, I was on nerve pain medication for months. It was called gabapentin. The medicine interferes with the same receptors as ketamine, so it can eliminate the visions and impact the antidepressant benefits. Benzodiazepines like Xanax and Valium act in a similar way. If you are prescribed these medications, do not stop taking them without talking to your doctor. It can trigger a host of dangerous problems including seizures.

LATEST DIARY ENTRY, FROM 6/9

I screwed up. My 2,700mg per day gabapentin dose from my surgeries earlier this year is competing for the same NMDA receptor as the ketamine. Although I got the medicine just fine, I wasn't able to see much in terms of visions.

I could only faintly make out different things here and there. It was like being blind.

Midway, I decided that I would feel my way around with my heart since I couldn't see. Sounds odd when I write it, but it seemed normal at the time. I started to view myself in the third person, checking myself into treatment for the first time. My heart broke for that young man. My heart just broke for him. I was seeing and feeling him in the third person and my eyes teared up as I mourned for him.

People don't understand the heartbreak that exists there, I'm guessing because the addict's ego casts a veil over the addiction that can't be pierced. Nobody knows the pain because he is too afraid to show it. I was too afraid to show it.

I'm in a deep meditative state again, but without the breath-work. Some of my best thinking is done here, free from chatter and the voice on my shoulder. It comes at a material cost — but the material world is nothing but a blip on the radar compared to this other place. It doesn't matter because there you exist without the self. I am there, but the social framework for what makes me myself is gone, including monetary status. All that's left is the heart, and unfiltered thinking.

It's impossible to lie to yourself here. Perhaps that's why it is so effective for solving problems.

I can't work right now because my right hand is still numb from surgery. I can't feel the keys on my laptop ... but it doesn't matter. I just need to do the right thing, and take care of myself physically, emotionally, and spiritually.

If I align my work with who I am inside, then the monetary reward naturally will come. I've proven this time and time again. If my work isn't in line with who I am, I get blocked and can't think. Frustration and stress sets in.

But on the flip side, if I do what does align with who I am ... work isn't work, it's simpler. It becomes light, using the momentum of, "This is me. This is my purpose."

Even though I didn't see much today, I feel very lucky. And realigned. Tomorrow, when my uncle comes over to talk about our disagreements from eight weeks ago, I'll meet him with understanding and compassion. Even though my family struggles with showing me the same, it is still the most efficient problem solver. FTW.

REFERENCES

https://www.ncbi.nlm.nih.gov/pmc/articles/PMC5126726/

https://www.nber.org/digest/sep14/patent-expiration-and-pharmaceutical-prices

https://www.accessdata.fda.gov/drugsatfda_docs/nda/2019/211243Orig1s000ClinPharmR.pdf

https://www.psychologytoday.com/us/blog/two-takes-depression/201904/ketamine-vs-esketamine-depression

https://www.npr.org/sections/health-shots/2019/04/11/712295937/ketamine-may-relieve-depression-by-repairing-damaged-brain-circuits

https://www.ncbi.nlm.nih.gov/books/NBK470357/

https://www.ichelp.org/new-research-shows-how-ketamine-abuse-causes-bladder-damage/

https://www.science.org/doi/full/10.1126/science.aat8078

https://psychedelicinvest.com/how-many-different-types-of-psychedelic-mushrooms-are-there/

https://pubmed.ncbi.nlm.nih.gov/31132970/

https://www.psychedelicsinrecovery.org/wp-content/uploads/2019/04/Distilled-Spirits-excerpt.pdf

https://www.cancer.gov/publications/dictionaries/cancer-terms/def/schedule-i-drug

https://www.sondermind.com/private-practice/phq9-overview

https://pubmed.ncbi.nlm.nih.gov/31532029/

https://www.sciencedirect.com/topics/neuroscience/default-mode-network#:~:text=The%20default%20mode%20network%20(DMN,measurable%20with%20the%20fMRI%20technique.

https://www.researchgate.net/publication/345260212_Ketamine_can_be_produced_by_Pochonia_chlamydosporia_an_old_molecule_and_a_new_anthelmintic

https://elifesciences.org/articles/59784

https://pubmed.ncbi.nlm.nih.gov/25877327/

https://www.wbur.org/news/2018/09/10/ibogaine-psychedelic-opioid-misuse-therapy

AUTHOR'S NOTE

When I first had the idea of writing a book, I was 30. I never took it seriously and it was always a "maybe one day" idea. At the very least, I thought, I'd start keeping a diary of sorts when I learned something new or of value.

When the voice inside told me to write this book, I immediately ignored it. There were too many risks — risks of time, money, and "reputation." I kept working on my e-commerce business — Youtube ads are a booming business right now.

But there was one problem ... every time I tried to work on my ad business, my neck would hurt ... bad. I literally couldn't do it. After trying and failing multiple variables (stand up desk, etc.) I finally gave in and started writing. And just like that, my neck stopped bothering me and I was able to work. Hmmm, funny how that works. ...

I hope my book inspires you, helps reveal options, etc. Do authors even make money? I don't think many do - the point was always to help others. After breaking my back my income halted with my inability to type. I say this not to make you feel bad for me ... don't.

Instead of focusing on generating a profit, I hope to spread the message of the psychedelic approach to mental health that has helped me in such dramatic ways. This takes advertising money and online promotion.

How can you help me accomplish that? It's simple, easy, and free. Leave a review on the platform you purchased it from. That simple act will help boost the listing and spread the message to others that wouldn't have otherwise known about these new treatment options.

I will keep this section as a placeholder to provide you a link to the amazon listing. Thank you for reading, and supporting my message by leaving a review! (placeholder for link)

PS: Keep an eye out for my next book, which is the second memoir in this 2 book series where I share dramatic experiences with ibogaine for opiate use disorder, psilocybin, and ayahuasca ... coming 2023.

RESOURCES

For those on the journey of healing and self-development, here are some resources to consider.

***Keynote speaking**, please message me directly on Instagram @dlamar_1

*DO NOT MISS my **FREE psychedelic resources guide**, delivered to your phone!

Scan the QR code to access...

- Top Secret Psychedelic Treatment Playlists
- Psychedelic Integration Checklist & Interactive Journal

- Discounted Eye Masks
- Treatment Provider Discounts ... and MORE!

Or visit https://rainmedia.co/resources

*Join Me & Understanding Ketamine on Patreon.

Scan the QR code to access...

- Exclusive personal content
- Treatment resources and reviews on providers worldwide
- Responsible psychedelic discussion
- Access to our community
- Releases of never-before-seen chapters from my upcoming book.

*Interested in **legal psychedelic treatments** but not sure where to start? Take our FREE quiz (coming soon) and we will put you in touch with a qualified professional who can help.

Or visit https://patreon.com/DLamar

*Do you or a loved one need help sourcing...

- **Ketamine providers** (cash only)

OR

- **Traditional substance abuse treatment**, or **therapy** (private insurance or cash pay)

Email info@rainmedia.co, or take the FREE quiz on www.rainmedia.co (coming soon).

*For help with **e-commerce, business, and personal development coaching**, apply on www.rainmedia.co or message me directly on Instagram @dlamar_1

Please note, 1-on-1 coaching is not a fit for everyone, nor is it inexpensive. I look forward to finding out if it is a good fit for you!

*Follow me on...

Instagram.com @dlamar_1

Patreon.com @dlamar

Manufactured by Amazon.ca
Acheson, AB